KT-222-553

When a Child has Cancer

NAPIER UNIVERSITY LIS

When a Child has Cancer

Ann Faulkner
Professor in Communication Studies at Sheffield University Medical School and
Deputy Director at Trent Palliative Care Centre

Gillian Peace
Research Associate

and

Catherine O'Keeffe
Research Associate

LIBRARY
LOTHIAN COLLEGE OF HEALTH STUDIES
13 CREWE ROAD SOUTH
EDINBURGH
EH4 2LD

CHAPMAN & HALL
London · Glasgow · Weinheim · New York · Tokyo · Melbourne · Madras

Published by Chapman & Hall, 2–6 Boundary Row, London SE1 8HN, UK

Chapman & Hall, 2–6 Boundary Row, London SE1 8HN, UK

Blackie Academic & Professional, Wester Cleddens Road, Bishopbriggs, Glasgow G64 2NZ, UK

Chapman & Hall GmbH, Pappelallee 3, 69469 Weinheim, Germany

Chapman & Hall USA, One Penn Plaza, 41st Floor, New York NY 10119, USA

Chapman & Hall Japan, ITP-Japan, Kyowa Building, 3F, 2-2-1 Hirakawacho, Chiyoda-ku, Tokyo 102, Japan

Chapman & Hall Australia, Thomas Nelson Australia, 102 Dodds Street, South Melbourne, Victoria 3205, Australia

Chapman & Hall India, R. Seshadri, 32 Second Main Road, CIT East, Madras 600 035, India

Distributed in the USA and Canada by Singular Publishing Group Inc., 4284 41st Street, San Diego, California 92105

First edition 1995

© 1995 Ann Faulkner, Gillian Peace and Catherine O'Keeffe

Typeset in 10/12pt Times by Saxon Graphics Ltd, Derby
Printed in Great Britain by St. Edmundsbury Press, Bury St. Edmunds, Suffolk

ISBN 0 412 59260 0 1 56593 331 1

Apart from any fair dealing for the purposes of research or private study, or criticism or review, as permitted under the UK Copyright Designs and Patents Act, 1988, this publication may not be reproduced, stored, or transmitted, in any form or by any means, without the prior permission in writing of the publishers, or in the case of reprographic reproduction only in accordance with the terms of the licences issued by the Copyright Licensing Agency in the UK, or in accordance with the terms of licences issued by the appropriate Reproduction Rights Organization outside the UK. Enquiries concerning reproduction outside the terms stated here should be sent to the publishers at the London address printed on this page.

The publisher makes no representation, express or implied, with regard to the accuracy of the information contained in this book and cannot accept any legal responsibility or liability for any errors or omissions that may be made.

A catalogue record for this book is available from the British Library

Library of Congress Catalog Card Number: 95–67591

∞ Printed on permanent acid-free text paper, manufactured in accordance with ANSI/NISO Z39 48-1992 and ANSI/NISO Z39. 48-1984 (Permanence of Paper).

Contents

Preface

This book is about a research project on the effect of childhood cancer on both the patient and other family members. As a team we were impressed with the openness of all those that we interviewed and with their willingness to share their thoughts and feelings with us.

The material we gathered was so rich and gave such clear messages about the effects of childhood cancer that we decided to write it up in this book so that we can share both the positive and negative aspects, from a number of perspectives, including those of the formal carers in both hospital and community.

By drawing on past research and exploring our interactions with the families in our study, we hope to leave our readers with some views on how members of a family, where a child has cancer, can be further helped and supported while they adapt to a life-threatening illness and an uncertain future.

Ann Faulkner
Gillian Peace
Catherine O'Keeffe

Acknowledgements

This study would not have been possible without the help and support of a number of colleagues. Professor Eric Wilkes suggested the study, Professor David Clark had input to the original negotiations and design, and Dr Mary Gerrard kindly gave us access to the families in the study and support and advice along the way.

We would also like to express our gratitude to the families who agreed to take part in this study, and our professional colleagues who care for those families. Without exception they were prepared to share their views and experiences of being involved in a very difficult situation.

Finally, we would like to thank our colleagues at Trent Palliative Care Centre for their help and support, especially Pauline Hutchinson who typed, and re-typed (!) the final manuscript.

Ann Faulkner
Gillian Peace
Catherine O'Keefe

Introduction

The experience of coping with a life-threatening illness in a child must be one of the most distressing life events that a family has to face. Due to advances in medicine, both in prevention and treatment, fewer children die as a result of illness than in the past. In the field of childhood cancer the prognosis has improved dramatically (Birch *et al.*, 1988; Stiller, 1993). An improved diagnosis, however, does not reduce the emotional impact on families. Instead they face a different kind of anguish. No longer is the outcome certain death but rather the prospect of uncertainty about future health and survival – a prospect which has aptly been described as living with the 'Damocles syndrome' (Eisenberg, 1981).

The Greek myth tells of Damocles, flatterer of Dionysius, the lover of all good things in life, who sat at a banquet with a sword suspended above his head by a single hair to impress upon him the precariousness of happiness. The human condition – the inescapable confrontation with the threat of tragedy – is the subject matter of much Greek drama. Ronald Harwood (1984) has commented that the Greek dramatists knew life's pains and terrors and man's dark and irrational responses to it but they also believed that life was to be enjoyed and made use of the healing power of laughter. Out of this paradox came the impetus to create 'something for the living even out of death [or the threat of death]' – an impetus that has generated many creative achievements through the ages. The 'pains and terrors' are evident in the stories told by the families in this book. At the same time many of their experiences reflect the creative and positive forces that can transform and transcend the darkness which most families feel permeates their lives when they first hear that their child has cancer.

BACKGROUND TO THE STUDY

There was a need to explore the new challenges to families and carers in this field not only because of the improved prognosis for children with cancer. Society has changed in other ways which affect how families cope with this experience. The rise in the number of marriages which break up, resulting in more single parents and more reconstituted families, means that family relationships are more complex. Increasingly family members live geographically distant from each other reducing the opportunity for mutual support. Many communities are multiracial and multicultural adding further to the changing demands on professionals involved in the care of child and family.

Before embarking on a study to investigate the psychosocial needs of families facing childhood cancer it was necessary to examine the position of research and current knowledge on the subject in the light of these changes. A literature review was undertaken.

Literature review

Four aspects of recent research were considered: the effects childhood cancer has on children and their families, the ways in which intervention can meet the resultant needs, the methodological difficulties encountered by researchers in this field and the ability of professionals to provide support.

The assessment of psychosocial effects has been approached from a number of directions. Four major routes can be identified, reflecting the multidimensional nature of a family's response and ability to cope with childhood cancer:

● the disease trajectory and its characteristics;
● the individual within the family;
● the family as a single unit;
● social and cultural influences.

Some aspects have had more attention than others. The list reflects the **evolution** and the **amount** of interest relating to each dimension. For example early literature focused on the dying child and preparation for death and bereavement. Later many studies examined individual and dyad responses such as the patient, siblings, parents, mother and patient. More recently there has been a growing awareness that it is the whole family which is profoundly affected by this experience and that professionals should regard the family as the unit of care. Social and cultural aspects have received the least attention.

Medical progress and influence has clearly affected the study approach. Firstly there is a continuing focus on the disease; changing from examining the child **dying of** cancer to the child and family **living with** cancer – moving from the perception of childhood cancer as a terminal to a chronic disease. Secondly the use of quantitative methods and psychometric scales predominates – features characteristic of the medical model. Thirdly these research tools have been used to measure pathological symptoms which are inappropriate when studying normal individuals under stress (Sourkes, 1987).

Before considering the effects and interventions in the context of these dimensions it is important to emphasize that such divisions are artificial and applied for the sake of clarity. In reality the way in which individuals respond to a crisis is influenced by factors originating from each of these dimensions.

THE DISEASE TRAJECTORY AND ITS CHARACTERISTICS

Effects

The most stressful times, for parents in particular, during the course of the illness are when they are told the diagnosis, the days immediately afterwards before treatment begins and the first relapse after treatment. Many believe the diagnosis means death, despite the improved prognosis, and suffer anticipatory mourning. With each relapse the threat of loss resurfaces and intensifies with the narrowing of hope (Maguire, 1983; Van Dongen-Melman and Sanders-Wouldstra, 1986; Geen, 1990; Macaskill and Monach, 1990).

The treatment period presents different problems. There are those associated with hospitalization. The child feels a sense of alienation and isolation as a result of being separated from home and family members and a loss of independence and control (Cartwright, 1983). Parents too feel a loss of control in terms of health professionals taking over parental responsibilities (Black and Wood, 1989; Geen, 1990). Problems associated with the treatment programme, for the patient and family members, can include coping with the physical discomfort of side effects which can be worse than the symptoms of the disease. The more complex the treatment the more the child is affected (Katz, 1980). There can also be distressing visible body changes some of which may be irreversible. But overshadowing all these possible concerns is the fact that a cure cannot be guaranteed.

Transition from hospital to home is a time when the family may feel particularly vulnerable, even abandoned, without the support of health professionals (Macaskill and Monach, 1990). There are many difficulties adjusting to normal life when recurrence of the disease is a constant threat (Koocher, 1984). Various studies have shown that families never return to 'normal' and are permanently changed by the experience (Ross-Alaolmolki, 1986; Schuler *et al.*, 1985). Long term survivors face many difficulties even though they have been disease free for many years (Koocher and O'Malley, 1981; Wallace *et al.*, 1987). These factors are considered in more detail in later sections.

Intervention

Throughout the course of the disease it has been found that good communication is imperative between families, child and health professionals both in terms of offering support and giving information. Parents cope better if they are told their child's diagnosis of a life-threatening disease openly, directly, early and sympathetically, in privacy with both parents present (Carr-Gregg and White, 1985; Stein *et al.*, 1989). It is difficult to take everything in because of the shock and confusion. This leads to a need for information to be repeated and clarified. Conveying an honest, realistic outlook is considered the best approach. Presenting a 'rosy' or over-optimistic view of the prognosis undermines rather than supports the parents' care (Culling, 1988; Arnfield, 1990; Macaskill and Monach, 1990).

Myra Bluebond-Langer's work (1990) suggests that experience is more critical than age in a child's understanding of illness. This supports the growing awareness that even very young children are able to understand the nature and implications of a serious illness. With this awareness has come a greater acceptance of the concept of children's rights and the importance of their involvement in the decision making process (Harboard *et al.*, 1987; Susman, Dorn and Fletcher, 1987; Moore and Ruccione, 1989). There is evidence that children who are told their diagnosis earlier and are given an opportunity to discuss it show better psychosocial adjustment than others (Slavin *et al.*, 1982).

During the period of diagnostic tests and treatment there is a need for adequate preparation of the child and for adequate information for the whole family. Anticipatory fears and phobias are common in children as they have to cope with repeated painful procedures and several courses of treatment. Skilful, planned preparation can help alleviate them (Culling, 1988; Casey, 1990). Some studies have emphasized that focusing on details at this time, rather than on the more general 'tragic' picture, can help parents cope better (Shapiro, 1983). Including parents in the care of their child whilst in hospital can also enhance their sense of control over the situation (Geen, 1990).

Provision of psychosocial support for the whole family is widely considered essential. But questions remain:

● Do all families need it?
● Is it effective in reducing the stress experienced by families?
● At what stage is it most needed?
● In what form is it most beneficial – targeting the individual, group or family unit, and pitched at a superficial or in-depth level?

THE INDIVIDUAL WITHIN THE FAMILY

The majority of studies have approached the subject of psychosocial factors in childhood cancer by examining the effects and coping mechanisms of individuals or dyads within the family. It is clear from this work that, despite the need for health professionals to be aware of the family functioning as a unit, each member of the family may have specific needs requiring individually tailored intervention.

One branch of family relationships has received little attention – the grandparents. They are frequently significant members of the family and have a double burden seeing their grandchild and their child in pain (Geen, 1990). Members of the family whose experiences have been explored include the child with cancer, parents and siblings.

The Child with Cancer

Most studies investigating the effects on children with cancer do not obtain the view of the child, and those that have are mainly retrospective (Carr-Gregg and White, 1985; Moore and Ruccione, 1989). There is little information, other than anecdotal, which shows how the child feels at the time of experiencing the various stages and procedures he or she has to endure.

Further, trying to establish levels of seriousness of psychosocial disturbance is a complex matter. Most studies examine the patient at one point in the illness not throughout. Correcting this weakness in method by the use of a longitudinal study would be difficult however, because of the unpredictable course of the disease and its potential disruption of important developmental stages during childhood. A further weakness found in some studies is that adult measurement tools geared to a psychologically disturbed population have been adapted for use on children and interpreted by adults (Koocher *et al.*, 1980; Spinetta and Deasy-Spinetta, 1981). The use of these tools places some doubt on the accuracy of the results achieved.

Effects

Despite these methodological weaknesses there is some consistency of view. Regardless of age or cognitive development most children with cancer realise that it is no ordinary illness. Some may blame themselves and see it as a punishment. The younger child appears more concerned about body integrity than survival. The adolescent is more concerned about change in body image, disruption to everyday living and the fulfilment of expected goals in relation to career, marriage or having a family (Spinetta and Deasy-Spinetta, 1981; Carr-Gregg and White, 1985). It seems the younger the child at onset and the shorter the length of treatment, the fewer the difficulties in emotional adjustment (Culling, 1988). However, many feel isolated and lonely in hospital, fearful of the diagnostic and treatment procedures and their side effects and the possibility of relapse. The child's distress is sometimes expressed through behavioural problems, sometimes through emotional disturbances. Depression, regression, withdrawal, temper tantrums and sleep disturbances are not uncommon (Van Dongen-Melman and Sanders-Wouldstra, 1986; Arnfield, 1990).

Intervention

The general trend in helping the child cope is through guiding the parents to support him or her through open and honest communication concerning the diagnosis, treatment and prognosis. Children who learn of their diagnosis in this way at an early stage adjust better. If they are told later they may feel betrayed, shocked and more fearful of the consequences (Slavin *et al.*, 1982). Also, if information is inadequate, children develop their own views built on fantasy or what they glean from their parents' reactions which may be maladaptive and mirrored in the child. If there is open and honest communication there is less likelihood of emotional and behavioural disturbances (Geen, 1990).

How information is conveyed to children is important. It is necessary to assess the child's cognitive development, to communicate in an age-appropriate manner and to re-explain over time in a more sophisticated manner as the child's cognitive ability develops (Susman, Dorn and Fletcher, 1987). Culling (1988) has emphasized that children find it difficult to put their fears into words and need the opportunity to express them through play, painting or drawing. Whilst some children clearly do have difficulties in talking, it is interesting to note that one study found that younger girls – who were the most inquisitive and talkative – appeared least anxious (Katz, Kellerman and Siegel, 1980). If a health professional skilled in communication with children were to encourage the natural inquisitiveness of most children in relation to aspects of their illness there could be benefit in terms of improved psychosocial adjustment. This has implications for those researchers investigating the child's perspective, a previously neglected area possibly because of fears that the child might be harmed through talking about his or her illness.

The greatest support to the ill child should be the family. However, an important source which could be overlooked is the child's peer group. Patient groups can be helpful and the patient's friends should be encouraged to visit in hospital (Geen, 1990). Maintaining links with school both with teachers and peers and continuing school work with the help of the hospital teacher establishes a sense of normality, prevents impairment of emotional and intellectual development caused by prolonged hospitalization and facilitates transition back to school after discharge.

Parents

The majority of studies have interviewed parents together or concentrated on the mother/child dyad. Subsequently there is little reliable information on the differences of experience or differential coping between mothers and fathers. Yet one study has shown the profound effect the child's illness has had on fathers (Fife, 1980). The needs of fathers have, in general, been ignored or assigned a peripheral role by health professionals. The difficulty about the data which follows is that it is impossible to differentiate between the perspectives of mothers and fathers except where the mother only has been interviewed. This section, therefore, refers to both parents as though they had a single perspective, which cannot always be assumed.

Effects

With the improved prognosis of childhood cancer, parents have the immensely painful task of balancing an awareness of the possibility of death with a realistic hope of their child's survival (Koocher and O'Malley, 1981). This situation appears to be more difficult to handle for some than the prospect of certain death of their child even following apparently successful treatment (Bartholome, 1978; Spinetta and Deasy-Spinetta, 1981). For example if the child who has been realistically mourned survives there can be problems of reintegration of the child into the family requiring professional help (Van Dongen-Melman and Sanders-Woudstra, 1986). These findings highlight an interesting discrepancy between parents and children: parents worry about the future, 'will my child die?'. Children worry about the present, 'that looks a huge needle, it's going to hurt' (Levenson et al., 1983; Spinetta, 1984). The effects on parents besides grief, fear and anxiety, can include guilt, blame, denial of the reality of the situation, flights into activity, hostility towards health professionals and feelings of being overwhelmed by the child's care (Shapiro, 1983).

This heavy emotional burden can affect parents' attitudes to parenting. Commonly parents are over-protective, over-indulge the child and do not want their child told the diagnosis (Van Dongen-Melman and Sanders-Woudstra, 1986; Geen, 1990). They may subsequently feel a debt of guilt concerning the siblings because the family routine has revolved around the patient. Maguire (1983) doubts if it is ever possible to treat a child with cancer 'normally' again. Some parents (and patients too) may feel their authority is taken over by health professionals, challenging their competence. At the same time extra demands are made on parenting skills in terms of caring, supporting, talking about the diagnosis and its implications and preparing the child for treatment.

In addition to having to cope with their own and their child's suffering and the total disruption to family life, there are practical difficulties including increased costs incurred through prolonged and repeated hospital visits and possible loss of income due to time off work to devote to the child's care (Cairns et al., 1981; Lansky et al., 1983).

There has been considerable focus on marital breakdown to assess how parents cope under such pressures. Yet it has been shown that divorce rates have not increased as a result of childhood cancer, although difficulties which already existed tend to be exacerbated (Kaplan et al., 1973; Lansky et al., 1978; Maguire et al., 1979; Peck, 1979). There are conflicting opinions as to whether the experience can have positive effects on the marriage. Lansky and colleagues (1978) conclude that couples are not brought closer together. However Macaskill and Monach (1990) report that several of their respondents said that despite the little time they had together due to dividing care between patient and siblings they felt closer as a result of the illness.

Intervention

Parents can be helped in a number of ways. The staff/parent relationship is considered crucial both for parent and child:

● to enhance opportunities to discuss information given, to talk about feelings,

acknowledge the normality of them and deal with issues of guilt and blame either in peer groups or individually;
- to encourage taking the role of caretaker rather than guest while the child is in hospital;
- to create as normal an environment as possible both during and after treatment;
- to help and advise open communication;
- to promote a realistic view of the future;
- to appraise practical needs particularly regarding financial aspects (Shapiro, 1983; Culling, 1988; Stein *et al.*, 1989; Evans, 1990; Macaskill and Monach, 1990).

There is an important implication for intervention highlighted by Culling (1988). Some parents are apparently reluctant to admit to stress, and they perceive social workers as helpful in relation to financial but not for emotional problems. This puts the onus on health professionals to assess needs actively and elicit individual problems; skills which Maguire in two studies (1983; 1984) has found are frequently deficient. This is not because children are involved, as deficiencies have been found in other areas of care.

Siblings

Most studies concerning siblings have been retrospective and earlier ones are based on observations of parents rather than allowing siblings to speak for themselves. It is particularly important to explore the psychosocial impact on siblings, firstly because it is they who will live the longest with the memories and concerns related to the disease. Secondly because it appears that siblings suffer more than patients in terms of unattended emotional needs (Spinetta, 1981; Sourkes, 1987).

Effects

A recent study divided the problems of siblings into three:

- those related to the disruption of family relationships such as the sense of isolation, loneliness, alienation and confusion;
- those related to the focus of attention on the ill child such as anger, resentment, guilt, lack of power, jealousy and rivalry;
- those related to concern for their own health and the safety of their parents (Martinson *et al.*, 1990)

As with the ill child, the way in which siblings express themselves is dependent, in part, on the developmental stage reached. They may show their feelings through maladaptive behaviour such as withdrawal, enuresis, persistent abdominal pain or school problems. Infant and toddler siblings are thought to be at highest risk since they are unable to verbalize. They interpret family changes as parental rejection. Older siblings may take on the role of caretaker and use this as a defence against the resentment they feel (Spinetta, 1981; Carr-Gregg and White, 1985; Sourkes, 1987; Martinson et al., 1990).

Intervention

Most sibling problems are thought to be due to the over-protective approach adopted by parents (and in the past by health professionals) and closed communication patterns within the family. A cohesive family makes it easier for a sibling to adapt positively (Asada, 1987). Siblings, therefore, benefit from open, honest communication, clear, age-appropriate information and involvement in the ill child's care. These strategies lessen resentment, jealousy, fantasies and fears of contagion, guilt and blame (Culling, 1988; Geen, 1990). Involvement with the ill child's treatment and encouragement to be with the family and meet hospital and clinic staff help resolve the strain of separation and fantasies about the hospitalized child (Geen, 1990; Martinson et al., 1990). Geen also points out that a supported sibling can contribute to the support of the patient, underlining the importance of the ill child's peer group.

Just as parents are reluctant to admit stress, siblings do not always share their anxieties because they do not want to increase their parents' worries (Culling, 1988). Active intervention seems necessary. Group meetings can be useful (although one study emphasizes they are not suitable for all children) in providing peer group support, information about the disease, and the opportunity to express feelings and ask questions away from the rest of the family and the hospital ward (Kellerman et al., 1980; Stone, 1993).

Research in general in this field has tended to highlight only negative aspects. Gains, however, have been identified in relation to siblings besides the giving of mutual support, for example an increase in empathy for parents' needs, in closeness and respect for the ill sibling, and having to grow up more quickly (Iles, 1979). The latter, however, could equally be seen as negative in the sense of loss of carefree childhood.

The Family as a Single Unit

As research in this field has evolved there has been a gradual realization of the need to focus on the family as the relevant unit of care. In the context of paediatric care generally, Almond and colleagues have put it simply: 'the family is the patient' (Almond, Buckman and Gofman, 1979). Few studies have used a methodology which supports this maxim however. It has been argued that this is for ease of survey and that interconnections between child and family have been shown (Van Dongen-Melman and Sanders-Woudstra, 1986). Yet a family focus is appropriate for a number of reasons which become evident when it is seen how a family responds to this crisis.

Effects

Firstly, family communicating patterns appear to be critical in determining how well the family cope with the illness. A 'web of silence' can mask feelings of depression, denial, guilt, anxiety about the future and cause isolation of individual family members and separation from the outside world (Shapiro, 1983; Black and Wood, 1989).

Secondly, focusing on the family as a social system under severe stress allows for a broader assessment of strengths and weaknesses rather than concentrating for example on marital disharmony or divorce rates (Carr-Gregg and White, 1985). It is clear from the section above that childhood cancer causes disruption to **all** family relationships and to **each** member's whole way of life. The main reasons for this disruption are because of the life-threatening nature of the disease, the uncertainty of outcome and because of prolonged and repeated hospitalization which, due to increased centralization and the specialized nature of treatment, can be in units situated many miles from the family home.

The third reason why a family focus is appropriate is that the most accessible and significant sources of support are embedded in relationships with family members. The Royal College of Nursing has defined **the family** as the child's primary support group in his or her life. The significance of this is evident from a study which showed that a family's adverse response had a worse psychological effect on the child than the 'menace' of the disease itself (Gutton, 1978). Also the way families cope and the nature of the support given to supplement family resources depends on various 'family' factors – its structure, parenting style, and philosophy, its past history and concurrent problems (Fife, Norton and Groom, 1987; Kalnins *et al.*, 1980; Marky, 1982).

Fourthly, it has been noted that adaptive coping mechanisms can have conflicting results, as for example when parents' use of denial may reduce their own fear but restrict their perception of the needs of the rest of the family (Desmond, 1980). If there is a lack of understanding of the interactive nature of family relationships the significance of such differential coping might be underestimated.

Intervention

There are many aspects to do with the family unit which cannot be changed either because they are rooted in past experience, such as separation or divorce, or for practical reasons, such as the distance between the family home and the specialist hospital. However, changes in 'parenting style' and 'philosophy' are more accessible to professional influence. The evidence presented in previous sections shows that the families who are able to communicate effectively with each other, where the 'parenting style' could be described as open, appear to cope better. This is an area where professionals can strengthen family coping skills (Jenkins, 1989). Families can be encouraged to talk to each other about their fears and feelings to counteract isolation and gain strength by facing difficulties together. Culling (1988) has also suggested that expressing appropriate feelings without inhibitions helps people adapt to the reality of the situation. Counselling, or if necessary family therapy, can facilitate this process and can be particularly helpful where there are barriers to communication such as in denial, differential coping and conflict between parents (Macaskill and Monach, 1990).

Adequate information offered to all members of the family by health professionals, both in verbal and written form, is a key factor in helping families cope. However, several studies emphasize that some families may not be able to take in the information, some feel 'overawed', others feel 'put down', and others that the doctor is too busy to answer their questions. Moreover some may not believe what they are told (Shapiro, 1983; Evans, 1990). This highlights the importance of selecting the most appropriate person to give information – a person the family can trust and one who has time for discussion and clarification and the skills to elicit concerns specific to the individual family.

Clearly these are not the only ways of helping families cope. A thorough assessment of family factors including coping resources and responses, past history and concurrent stresses should open up areas of intervention whereby families can be supported. Addressing practical factors such as increased costs due to the illness can also enhance coping (Carr-Gregg and White, 1985). Shapiro (1983) is one of the few writers who has approached the subject of coping on the family level. She suggests the key areas to work on are helping families to live with continuing uncertainty and to build on positive aspects of relationships both within and outside the family.

The disruption to the family as a result of childhood cancer can be counteracted by efforts made to provide as normal an environment as possible. In hospital this is clearly difficult, however a family can be enabled to take active care of the child. This reduces the sense of loss of control felt by parents, isolation felt by the patient and lack of involvement felt by siblings. The use of a primary nurse can help build up trust with both child and family and the provision of a place within the hospital complex where a family can be alone together has been recommended (Geen, 1990).

To encourage the 'loosening of dependency on the hospital' after discharge, health professionals can visit families in their home, placing an emphasis on return to normal life, assisting in transition back to school and the care of the primary health team, by liaising with and providing appropriate information to teachers, the general practitioner and community nurses. However these efforts are to some extent jeopardized by the necessary return to hospital for check ups (Culling, 1988).

Social and Cultural Influences

Adherents of family systems theory stress the significance of viewing the family as part of a 'whole', that is of a society or culture (Schulz, 1984). Others have noted how people's perceptions of children change over time and emphasize the importance of seeing the family within the context of modern society (Aries, 1960). Evidence from a number of studies suggests that a family's cultural, social and educational background and their relationship with the society and environment in which they live all have an influence on how they respond to the impact of childhood cancer (Koocher and O'Malley, 1981; Shapiro, 1983; Spinetta, 1984), yet there are few studies which openly acknowledge this.

Effects

One of the recurrent factors to emerge is that the subject of cancer evokes strong feelings in many people. Society's attitudes to cancer are often characterized by prejudice, stigma, a sense of helplessness, even phobia. Such adverse attitudes clearly affect how a family copes and add to the sense of vulnerability and isolation some feel (Geen, 1990; Macaskill and Monach, 1990). This isolation is exacerbated by changing social factors such as reduced family size, nuclear as opposed to extended families and increased geographical mobility which has reduced access to social support and made it more difficult for families to accept and cope with illness (Hirschfield and Krulik, 1985). Comaroff and Maguire (1981) have argued that advances in medicine can be ambiguous when seen in the light of such changes in modern society. Conversely the rise in living standards and improvements in communications counteract some of the effects of these demographic changes by allowing contacts to remain at a high level (Wilmott, 1986).

This discrepancy of views highlights the need to be alert to a family's financial circumstances – maintaining contact is costly. High economic status has been linked with the likelihood of successful adjustment. In a sample of 'affluent' families who needed considerable extra emotional support Macaskill and Monach (1990) commented: 'how much greater must be the need in families where coping resources are already stretched by their circumstances before the onset of the child's illness?' In a paper reviewing ten years on from the Black report of 1980, the conclusion reached is that social class differences in relation to morbidity and mortality are widening (Davey Smith, Bartley and Blane, 1990). This finding has been confirmed as a continuing trend by Phillimore, Beattie and Townsend (1994). There is clearly need for continued vigilance on this issue, since not only has it been shown that poorer people are more likely to suffer from ill health but also they have more difficulties in coping with the resultant problems.

A family's response to childhood cancer is in part influenced by their ethnic and cultural background. Patterns of communication, shown to be of importance in relation to adaptive coping, differ in families of different ethnic origin. For example Mexican and Vietnamese families tend to have more closed patterns of communication and apparently adapt with more difficulty (Spinetta, 1984). In some cultures the family has a particularly strong role. For these families the perceived 'takeover' of professional carers may cause problems (Flomenhaft, 1984).

Intervention

The scope for changing adverse social and cultural influences is limited for the majority of health professionals and in the case of cultural factors ethically unacceptable. Extra help whether attending to emotional, financial or practical needs is clearly necessary for those with low income or who come from a deprived environment; however changing attitudes is notoriously difficult and slow. Nevertheless education has a role to play to enlighten society and families about the changes and progress in cancer care and to alert health professionals to the needs of a changing, multicultural, multiracial, modern society.

One factor which can powerfully influence changes in attitudes is personal experience. The experience of childhood cancer has mostly been recorded in negative terms, however a few studies have reported positive aspects (Koocher and O'Malley, 1981; Kupst *et al.*, 1982). It is valuable to know the positive effects, not only because of the need to learn about making a life-threatening illness a major growth experience for the family, but also because the more widely these positive aspects are felt and shared the more quickly attitudes should change and the taboo, fear and stigma which still surrounds childhood cancer should lessen.

Most of this chapter has been devoted to identifying the psychosocial needs of individuals and families faced with childhood cancer and the interventions recommended to meet those needs. The question as to whether those needs are being met by health professionals is more difficult to answer, primarily because the major gap in research in this field is the lack of evaluation of intervention measures. It is not yet known either what forms of intervention, particularly in the provision of emotional support, help families cope best, or whether health professionals have the appropriate skills and resources to provide support (Maguire, 1983; Nicholson, 1990). Intervention has largely been based on clinical experience, 'intuition' and 'guesswork' (Culling, 1988; Casey, 1990). This omission is perhaps understandable in the light of the comment that the effectiveness of supportive measures is difficult to assess as so many factors are involved – if a family adapts well how do we know which intervention contributed most? And what is the meaning of support (Casey, 1990)?

Another aspect of effectiveness of intervention is the stressful nature of the work. It is widely acknowledged that stress affects the work performance of health professionals. They may become over-involved or detached and many are susceptible to burnout (Shubin, 1978; Storlie, 1979; Sepion, 1990). There is clearly a need for improved provision of education and training to equip staff to deliver effective and efficient care particularly in the area of assessment and eliciting a family's individual concerns together with adequate support and supervision for those working in such a demanding environment.

CONCLUSIONS

The changes in medical practice in the field of childhood cancer and in society generally impose even greater stresses on individuals and families faced with life-threatening illness in a child than previously. Despite the large amount of data available there are significant gaps in our knowledge, primarily because the majority of research in the area has been disease-related.

The lack of focus, in varying degrees, on the ill child's perspective at the time of diagnosis and treatment, on the separate and possibly differing perspectives of the mothers and fathers, on the siblings and grandparents, indicates that there is little known about family relationships and how they change over time in the effort to cope. There is also little understanding about how previous and concurrent experiences (not associated with the child's illness) affect these relationships. The whole process of investigation before diagnosis through treatment and adjustment to life back at home can take several years and much can happen in the meantime which influences the way families cope.

In an attempt to understand the changing needs of families facing childhood cancer, a study was designed to address some of the gaps in current research. The intention was to focus on the whole family as the unit of investigation with an awareness of both individual needs and the wider influences of culture and social environment. The planning and results of the study form the remainder of this book.

REFERENCES

Almond, B., Buckman, W. and Gofman, H.F. (1979) *The Family is the Patient – An Approach to Behavioural Pediatrics.* Mosby, London.

Aries, P. (1960) *Centuries of Childhood.* Penguin Books, Harmondsworth.

Arnfield, A. (1990) Common issues relating to diagnosis and treatment, in *The Child with Cancer – Nursing Care*, (ed J. Thompson) Scutari Press, London, pp. 31–47.

Asada, C.A. (1987) The identification of siblings of paediatric cancer patients at risk for maladaptive coping responses. *Dissertation Abstract International*, **(B)47**(8), 3507.

Bartholome, W.G. (1978) The shadow of childhood cancer and society's responsibilities, in *Proceedings of the National Conference on the Care of the Child Cancer Patient.* American Cancer Society, New York.

Birch, J.M., Marsden, H.B., Morris-Jones, P.H. *et al.* (1988) Improvements in survival from childhood cancer: results of a population based survey over 30 years. *British Medical Journal*, **296**, 1372–6.

Black, D. and Wood, D. (1989) Family therapy and life threatening illness in children or parents. *Palliative Medicine*, **3**, 113–18.

Bluebond-Langer, M., Perkel, D. and Goertzel, T. (1990) Children's knowledge of cancer and its treatment: the impact of an oncology camp experience. *Journal of Paediatrics*, **1162**, 207–14.

Cairns, N.U., Clark, G.M., Black, J. and Lansky, S.B. (1981) Childhood Cancer: nonmedical costs of the illness, in *Living with Childhood Cancer,* (eds J.J. Spinetta and P. Deasy-Spinetta), Mosby, St Louis, pp. 121–32.

Cairns, N.U., Clark, G.M., Smith, S.D. and Lansky, S.B. (1979) Adaptation of siblings to childhood malignancy. *Journal of Pediatrics*, **95**, 484–7.

Carr-Gregg, M.R.C. and White, L. (1985) The child with cancer: a psychological overview. *Medical Journal of Australia*, **143**, 503–6.

Cartwright, A. (1983) *Health Surveys in Practice and Potential*. Kings Fund, London.

Casey, A.M. (1990) The child and surgery, in *The Child with Cancer – Nursing Care*, (ed J. Thompson), Scutari Press, London, pp. 95–109.

Comaroff, J. and Maguire, P. (1981) Ambiguity and the search for meaning: childhood leukaemia in the modern clinical context. *Social Science in Medicine*, **15**, 115–23.

Culling, J.A. (1988) The psychological problems of families of children, in *The Supportive Care of the Child with Cancer,* (ed A. Oakhill), John Wright, Bristol, pp. 204–38.

Davey Smith, G., Bartley, M. and Blane, D. (1990) The Black report on socioeconomic inequalities in health 10 years on. *British Medical Journal*, **301**, 373–7.

Desmond, H. (1980) Two families: an intensive observational study, in *Psychological Aspects of Childhood Cancer*, (ed J. Kellerman), Charles C. Thomas, Springfield IL, pp. 100–127.

Eisenberg, L. (1981) Foreword, in *The Damocles Syndrome*, (eds G.P. Koocher and J.E. O'Malley), McGraw-Hill, New York, pp. xi–xv.

Evans, M. (1990) The child receiving chemotherapy, in *The Child with Cancer – Nursing Care*, (ed J. Thompson), Scutari Press, London, pp. 61–81.

Fife, B.L. (1980) Childhood cancer is a family crisis: a review. *Journal of Psychiatric Nursing*, **18**, 29–34.

Fife, B., Norton, J. and Groom, G. (1987) The family's adaptation to childhood leukaemia. *Social Science and Medicine*, **24**(2), 159–68.

Flomenhaft, K. (1984) Cross-cultural perspectives to childhood cancer, in *Childhood Cancer: Impact on the Family*, (eds A.E. Christ and K. Flomenhaft), Plenum Press, New York/London, pp. 159–76.

Geen, L.J. (1990) The family of the child with cancer, in *The Child with Cancer – Nursing Care*, (ed J. Thompson), Scutari Press, London, pp. 17–31.

Gutton, P. (1978) Psychopathology of the physically sick child. *Revue Neuropsychiat. Infant*, **26**, 471–6.

Harboard, M.G., Cross, D.G., Botica, F. and Martin, A.J. (1987) Children's understanding of cystic fibrosis. *Australian Paediatric Journal*, **23**, 241–4.

Harwood, R. (1984) *All the World's a Stage*. Secker and Warburg, London.

Hirschfield, M. and Krulik, T. (1985) Family caregiving to severely chronically ill children and the aged, in *Long-Term Care – Recent Advances in Nursing*, (ed K. King), Churchill Livingstone, London/Edinburgh, pp. 171–97.

Iles, J.P. (1979) Children with cancer: healthy siblings' perceptions during the illness experience. *Cancer Nursing*, **2**, 371–7.

Jenkins, H. (1989) The family and loss: a systems framework. *Palliative Medicine*, **3**, 97–104.

Kalnins, I.V., Churchill, M.P. and Terry, G.E. (1980) Concurrent stresses in families with a leukaemic child. *Journal of Pediatric Psychology*, **5**(1), 81–92.

Kaplan, B.M., Smith, A., Grobstein, R. and Fischerman, S.E. (1973) Family mediation of stress. *Social Work*, **18**, 60–69.

Katz, E.R. (1980) Illness impact and social reintegration, in *Psychological Aspects of Childhood Cancer*, (ed J. Kellerman), Charles C. Thomas, Springfield IL, pp. 14–46.

Katz, E.R., Kellerman, J. and Siegel, S. (1980) Behavioural distress in children undergoing medical procedures: developmental considerations. *Journal of Consulting and Clinical Psychology*, **48**, 356–65.

Kellerman, J., Zeltzer, L., Ettenberg, L. *et al.* (1980) Psychological effects of illness in adolescence – anxiety, self-esteem and perception of control. *Journal of Pediatrics*, **97**, 126–31.

Koocher, G.P. (1984) Coping with survivorship in childhood cancer: family problems, in *Childhood Cancer: Impact on the Family*, (eds A.E. Christ and K. Flomenhaft), Plenum Press, New York and London, pp. 201–3.

Koocher, G.P. and O'Malley, J.E. (1981) *The Damocles Syndrome*. McGraw-Hill, New York.

Koocher, G.P., O'Malley, J.E., Gogan, J.L. and Foster, D.J. (1980) Psychological adjustment among pediatric cancer survivors. *Journal of Child Psychology and Psychiatry*, **21**, 163–73.

Kupst, M.J., Schulman, J.L., Honig, G. *et al.* (1982) Family coping with childhood leukaemia: one year after the diagnosis. *Journal of Pediatric Psychology*, **7**, 157–74.

Lansky, S.B., Black, J.L. and Cairns, N.U. (1983) Childhood cancer: medical costs. *Cancer*, **52**, 762–6.

Lansky, S.B., Cairns, N.U., Hassanein, R. *et al.* (1978) Childhood cancer: parental discord and divorce. *Pediatrics*, **62**(2), 184–8.

Levenson, P.M., Copeland, D.R., Morrow, J.R. *et al.* (1983) Disparities in disease related perceptions of adolescent cancer patients and their parents. *Journal of Pediatric Psychology*, **8**(1), 33–5.

Macaskill, A. and Monach, J.H. (1990) Coping with childhood cancer: The case for longterm counselling help for patients and their families. *British Journal of Guidance and Counselling*, **18**(1), 13–26.

Maguire, G.P. (1983) The psychological sequelae of childhood leukaemia. *Recent Results in Cancer Research*, **88**, 47–56.

Maguire, P. (1984) Doctor–patient communication, in *Health Care and Human Behaviour*, (eds A. Matthews and A. Steptoe), Academic Press, London.

Maguire, G.P., Comaroff, J., Ramsell, P.J. and Morris Jones, P.H. (1979) Psychological and social problems in families of children with leukaemia, in *Topics in Paediatrics*, (ed P.H. Morris Jones), Pitman Medical, Tunbridge Wells.

Marky, I. (1982) Children with malignant disorders and their families: a study of the implications of the disease and its treatment on everyday life. *Acta Paediatrica Scandinavica*, **303**, 1–82.

Martinson, I.M., Gilliss, C., Colaizzo, D.C. *et al.* (1990) Impact of childhood cancer on healthy siblings. *Cancer Nursing*, **13**(3), 183–90.

Moore, I.M. and Ruccione, K. (1989) Challenges to conducting research with children with cancer. *Oncology Nursing Forum*, **16**(4), 587–9.

Nicholson, A. (1990) Childhood cancer – an overview, in *The Child with Cancer – Nursing Care*, (ed J. Thompson), Scutari Press, London, pp.1–17.

Peck, B. (1979) Effects of childhood cancer on long-term survivors and their families. *British Medical Journal*, **1**, 1327–9.

Phillimore, P., Beattie, A. and Townsend, P. (1994) Widening inequality in northern England, 1981–1991. *British Medical Journal*, **308**(6937), 1125–8.

Ross-Alaolmolki, K. (1986) Family functioning and coping in parents of children with leukaemia and parents of well school children. *Dissertation Abstract International* (**B**) **47**(4), 1736.

Schuler, D., Bakos, M., Zsambor, A. *et al.* (1985) Psychological problems in families of a child with cancer. *Medical and Pediatric Oncology*, **13**, 173–9.

Schulz, S.J. (1984) *Family Systems Therapy: An Integration.* Jason Aronsal, USA, pp. 53–76.

Sepion, B. (1990) Teamwork – caring for the child, the family and the staff, in *The Child with Cancer – Nursing Care*, (ed J. Thompson), Scutari Press, London, pp. 169–81.

Shapiro, J. (1983) Family reactions and coping strategies in response to the physically ill or the handicapped child: a review. *Social Science and Medicine*, **17**(14), 913–31.

Shubin, S. (1978) Burnout: the professional hazard you face. *Nursing*, **8**, 722.

Slavin, L.A., O'Malley, M.D., Koocher, G.P. and Foster, D.J. (1982) Communication of the cancer diagnosis to pediatric cancer patients: Impact on longterm adjustment. *American Journal of Psychiatry*, **139**(2), 179–83.

Sourkes, B.M. (1987) Siblings of the child with a life threatening illness. *Journal of Children in Contemporary Society*, **19**(3/4), 159–84.

Spinetta, J.J. (1981) Adjustment and adaptation in children with cancer: a 3 year study, in *Living with Childhood Cancer*, (eds J.J. Spinetta and P. Deasy-Spinetta), Mosby, St Louis, pp. 133–42.

Spinetta, J.J. (1984) Measurement of family function, communication and cultural effects. *Cancer*, **53**, 2230–7.

Spinetta, J.J. and Deasy-Spinetta, P. (1981) *Living with Childhood Cancer.* Mosby, St Louis.

Stein, A., Forrest, G.C., Woolley, H. and Baum, J.D. (1989) Life threatening illness and hospice care. *Archives of Disease in Childhood*, **64**, 697–702.

Stiller, C. (1993) Improvements in population in survival rates for childhood cancer in Britain 1980–1991. Paper presented at the International Association of Cancer Registries, London.

Stone, M. (1993) Lending an ear to the unheard: the role of support groups for siblings of children with cancer. *Child Health*, **1**(2), 54–8.

Storlie, F.J. (1979) Burnout: the elaboration of a concept. *American Journal of Nursing*, **79**, 2108–11.

Susman, E.J., Dorn, L.D. and Fletcher, J.C. (1987) Reasoning about illness in ill and healthy children and adolescents: Cognitive and emotional developmental aspects. *Journal of Developmental and Behavioural Pediatrics*, **8**(5), 266–73.

Van Dongen-Melman, J. and Sanders-Woudstra, J.A.R. (1986) Psychological aspects of childhood cancer: a review of the literature. *Journal of Child Psychology and Psychiatry*, **27**, 145–80.

Wallace, M.H., Reiter, P.B. and Pendergrass, T.W. (1987) Parents of long-term survivors of childhood cancer: a preliminary survey to characterize concerns and needs. *Oncology Nursing Forum*, **14**(3), 39–43.

Wilmott, P. (1986) *Social Networks: Informal Care and Public Policy.* Research Report 655, Policy Studies Institute, London.

LOTHIAN COLLEGE OF HEALTH STUDIES LIBRARY

2

Study Design and Methods

It can be seen from the literature that most of the studies of childhood cancer have focused on the disease from a medical perspective. Little insight has been shown on the experiences of individual family members and the family as a whole, and the question of how health professionals cope with the emotive nature of helping these families has not been considered.

The study described here was designed to explain some of the issues that had not previously been addressed. The study had three main aims:

- to develop a knowledge of the experiences of coping with malignant disease in childhood, from the perspectives of the child, key family members and professional carers;
- to develop a knowledge of the ways in which these experiences may change from pre-diagnosis, through diagnosis to adjustment to the changed situation within the 'normal' family life;
- to assess the feasibility of further systematic study of these experiences.

The first two aims focus on areas that do not appear to have been adequately addressed in previous research. The third aim raises the issue of how to conduct research in such a sensitive area.

The design and methods used will be examined in order to provide a clear outline of the study and some understanding of the complexities involved in this type of work. It will be presented on two levels. Firstly, two of the main methodological issues raised will be explored, namely the use of a qualitative approach and the ethical difficulties encountered. Secondly a description of the study will be given which will discuss how it was initiated and implemented.

METHODOLOGICAL ISSUES

Choice of approach: Qualitative or Quantitative?

When planning a research project it is essential to choose a method that is appropriate and will achieve the aims of the study. Choice can be influenced by what is considered to be acceptable practice within a particular field or subject area. In this study it was apparent that conventional approaches were inappropriate and would not enable the aims of the study to be achieved. As a result it was necessary to explore alternatives.

Medicine and health care has been dominated by a quantitative approach to research. This reflects the influence of science upon the development of the medical profession (Shiva, 1989). This influence has shaped the questions that medicine has asked and researched. Medical research has focused upon disease and its treatment. Quantitative research has enabled specific questions to be answered, such as the effect of a drug upon the course of a disease or the identification of the factors that are thought to cause an illness. This approach is particularly appropriate for the questions being asked. Quantitative research emphasizes objectivity, reliability, and validity. It enables relationships between variables to be examined and hypotheses to be tested. However this approach cannot be used to **explore** people's perceptions, experiences, and feelings.

The limitations of the medical model of health care have been recognized. In 1978, the World Health Organization (WHO) began to promote Primary Health Care which stresses the importance of focusing on health as opposed to illness (WHO, 1978). This change in emphasis has meant that questions being asked by health researchers are also changing. There is now much greater interest in how health is defined and how people live with the difficulties that illness can cause. Traditional methods of research which examine relationships between variables cannot address the complexities of the questions now being asked. What does it feel like to have a serious illness? How do families cope with the challenge of ill health? How does this differ from life before illness? The traditional research tools of medicine such as controlled trials or scales of psychiatric morbidity do not provide the information needed to answer these questions.

Eiser (1993) in a review of studies on children and chronic illness has pointed out that most of the research in this area has focused on psychopathology. This places emphasis on the psychiatric problems that people have in relation to coping as opposed to what it is like to live with illness. Bowling (1992) has conducted a critique of the scales and measures that are used to examine the psychological reaction of patients to illness. She states that, 'What is important is how the patient feels...'. However, the tools described focus on a medical agenda and aim to quantify feelings such as anxiety and depression. They do not explore patients' feelings as Bowling suggests they should. In this way scales and measures do not enable the experiences of those affected by illness to be examined from their perspectives. Simply asking patients how they feel and see their situation is not acknowledged as a way of finding out about psychological reactions.

Qualitative research is an approach developed in the field of sociology. Its focus is the exploration and understanding of issues that affect people's lives. From this understanding ideas and theories can be generated. Melia (1983) argues that the main advantage of qualitative research is its adaptability and flexibility. She suggests that it allows methods to be developed that enable the lives of people to be explored and greater understanding gained. Qualitative research encourages the researcher to study people's lives as they are, rather than as the researcher presumes they are. The beliefs of the researcher are not imposed upon the data gained from people they are studying, rather the researcher attempts to see the world from the point of view of the respondents.

The main criticism of this approach, often levied by those who are trained in traditional quantitative methods, is that it is seen to be anecdotal. It is argued that qualitative research is unreliable and invalid. Issues of reliability and validity are not ignored in qualitative research, rather the emphasis is on understanding people's lives (Glazer and Strauss, 1967). Glazer and Strauss (1967) argue that it is the responsibility of the researcher to ensure that themes and categories are derived directly from the data and reflect the perceptions of the respondents. Inevitably factors beyond the control of the researchers will influence the way they interpret data. Factors which appear to bias the data should be acknowledged. If a systematic approach is used in qualitative research, bias can be explored and used to the advantage of the study. Bias was evident in two aspects of this study. Three people carried out the data collection. Although all three had received a similar training in terms of interview technique and shared a similar philosophy, individuality meant that there would be some differences in the way the interviews were conducted. Regular discussion between the team members meant that differences could be explored and used as a means of obtaining greater insight into the data and research process.

The second area of bias related to the sample of families interviewed which were selected at the specialist centre as 'the best families', thus apparently under-representing families who were not coping well. In fact the bias revealed the assumptions of a medical perspective since 15 out of the 19 families described themselves as having difficulties for which extra intervention could have been appropriate. Again, in this example, bias once acknowledged is able to strengthen the insight that the study provides. In this sense Glazer and Strauss (1967) argue that whilst the reliability and validity of a research project must be considered, this process should facilitate rather than inhibit the generation of understanding, insight and ideas.

The aim of this study was to gain insight and understanding of the lives of families affected by childhood cancer. Qualitative research is thus an appropriate method to choose for the study. Interviewing family members and health professionals using a method that encourages people to share their perspectives, enables both their worlds and their lives to be explored. Asking people what happened, and how they felt about it, provides a wealth of data and the opportunity to identify and understand some of the issues that are important to those most affected by the illness. The method used ensured that the interviews were carried out in a sensitive and supportive manner. However asking people about emotional reactions to illness raised ethical issues.

ETHICAL ISSUES

Sieber (1992) suggests that there are three principles of ethical research: beneficence, respect and justice. Beneficence emphasizes that the outcome of research
should be of value and that it is carried out in a way that does not harm the
respondents. Respect stresses the need to protect respondents especially those
who are not autonomous such as children. Justice refers to the importance of
ensuring that the research is non exploitative. The issues of particular relevance
to this study were beneficence and respect. Avoiding harm and protecting the
vulnerable were seen to be of importance by the ethical committee. Interestingly
those who the ethical committee considered needed greatest protection were not
those that were found to be the most vulnerable.

Talking to people about feelings and talking to children raised most cause for
concern. Some health professionals believed that 'their' patients might be
damaged in some way by talking about their experiences. Children were
thought to be especially vulnerable. The ethical committee was concerned that
if children were interviewed about their experiences they may be unduly
distressed. Ethical approval was granted with two conditions: that children
under 16 would be interviewed by the project director who had considerable
experience in this area; and that children who were seen to be having difficulties
would be provided with expert psychiatric support. In terms of the design of the
project emphasis was placed on the preparation of the research team. The
researchers were trained in communication skills to ensure that interviews were
conducted sensitively, and accurately identified the perspectives of each participant in the study.

The training was based upon a model of assessment devised by Maguire and
Faulkner (1988). The model enables the interviewer to explore the participant's
experiences accurately and in a sensitive manner. The participant is given the
opportunity to express concerns and feelings. This approach emphasizes eliciting
the individual's concerns and feelings as opposed to simply answering questions
based on the interviewer's agenda. Although it is often cathartic to enable people
to share feelings in this way, it is essential that interviewers are able to 'lighten'
an interview so that participants are not left dwelling upon deeper emotions. The
model of assessment used contains several elements that facilitate this.
Negotiation is a central concept in this approach. Participants are encouraged to
disclose only those feelings that they feel able to share. If deeper feelings are
disclosed techniques such as summarizing concerns and screening for other areas
of concern are used to lighten the interview. Using this approach the interview
moves in and out of feelings so that the intensity of emotions does not become
too great. Negotiation about the length of the interview is important. Deciding on
a time frame helps to focus the interview and provides a guide for those taking
part because people often find it difficult to discuss such emotive issues.

Using this skilled approach the researchers were able to identify those individuals who were having difficulty coping. Five of the participants could have

benefited from medical intervention. A father, for example, of one of the adolescents in the retrospective group was found to be suffering from clinical depression. Only one of those in need of such help was a child. This child had a facial disfigurement as a result of her cancer. She was not coping with this and showed signs of depression. The ethical committee had placed great emphasis on protecting children and ensuring that they were adequately supported, but in doing so they were making three assumptions. Firstly they assumed that children would find it hard to talk about their illness. Secondly that they would need more support than adults, and thirdly that adults were unlikely to require extra specialist support. In fact the children in the study were much easier to talk to about cancer than the adults. They were very aware of the impact that the illness was having upon their parents and they tended to be more open and direct.

Whilst it needs to be acknowledged that children are vulnerable members of society assumptions should not be made about their ability to cope with illness and to express their feelings. Peace (1994) suggests that health professionals find talking to children particularly difficult due to a lack of skills to elicit the child's thoughts and feelings. As a result they often avoid discussing emotive issues. The techniques used to talk to children in this study were the same as those used with the adults. The effectiveness of this approach emphasizes the need to communicate with children in an open and honest manner.

The implications of the ethical dilemma confronted by this study are twofold. Firstly it suggests that the techniques used to talk to adults about illness can be effectively applied to talking with children. The successful application of these techniques developed by Maguire and Faulkner (1988) to research in this area indicates that future studies may benefit from developing a similar approach. Secondly assumptions should not be made upon a basis of age about the need for support when faced with a life-threatening illness. The adults, especially the parents, in this study were in much greater need of support than the children. This was not appreciated initially by the ethical committee and suggests that a more open approach is needed when assessing the potential impact of this type of research on those agreeing to participate.

DESCRIPTION OF THE STUDY

Background

The study was implemented at the Trent Palliative Care Centre. The centre is a relatively new research unit with a remit to develop education and research in palliative care. Recognition of the limitations of the work available in the area of children affected by life threatening illnesses led to consideration of the possibility of studying families affected by childhood cancer. A consultant paediatric oncologist at a regional centre for children with cancer expressed an interest and gave support to the project. The consultant initially introduced the researchers to a parents' organization, PACT. The parents were approached to ascertain their views on this type of work. They were very enthusiastic about the study, recognizing its value. Even at this stage the emotional intensity involved in studying this area was apparent. The group of parents in PACT spoke openly of their feelings and expressed their appreciation of having the opportunity to do so.

After ethical approval had been granted data collection began in 1991 and was completed in 1993. The study was designed as a pilot study. It was restricted to one regional specialist centre in the north of England. The specialist centre covered a geographical area with a radius of 80 miles.

The study was designed in three parts.

- **Retrospective**: nine families where the ill child had responded to treatment and had been in remission for between two and twelve years.
- **Prospective**: ten families where the ill child was still being treated or had recently finished treatment for cancer.
- **Health professionals**: 28 carers from both the regional centre and the community who had been involved with these families.

Individual family members in both the retrospective and prospective groups were interviewed in order to meet the first aim of gaining insight into different perspectives of family members and carers. The interviews with the health professionals provided the views of professional carers from both the hospital and community. The study was divided into retrospective and prospective groups to enable differences in experiences of living with childhood cancer over time to be explored, thus addressing the second aim. The third aim was achieved by evaluating how appropriate this methodology is for gaining insight into these experiences.

The 19 families in the study generated a total of 87 interviews. These included patients, fathers, mothers, siblings and where appropriate, grandmothers, grandfathers and aunts. The total number of refusals was six (see Table 2.1). The paediatric consultant oncologist who gave support to the study chose the families that were invited to take part, so they formed a sample of convenience.

Table 2.1 Family members in the study

	Prospective	Retrospective	Total
Patients	9	9	18
Fathers/stepfathers	9	8	17
Mothers	10	9	19
Brothers	5	1	6
Sisters	4	6	10
Grandfathers	4	2	6
Grandmothers	7	2	9
Aunts	2	0	2
Total	50	37	87

The health professionals interviewed included 18 doctors, nurses and social workers from the specialist paediatric oncology unit. Ten general practitioners were interviewed. These GPs were involved in the care of the families in the prospective group. The interviews involving community health workers were limited to these GPs. It was decided not to interview the GPs who cared for the retrospective group. This would have presented difficulties, for example, many would have moved. Similarly, community nurses such as health visitors were not interviewed for either group. Few had been directly involved in the care of these families. Those that had were no longer working in the area at the time of the study. Of the health professionals approached there were no refusals (Table 2.2).

Table 2.2   Health professionals in the study

General practitioners	10
Hospital consultants	2
Junior doctors	4
Qualified nurses *	8
Student nurses	2
Social workers *	2
Total	28

* All nurses and social workers interviewed were hospital based

Data Collection

Data collection began with the retrospective group. This helped to build the confidence of the clinicians in the ability of the research team to approach and interview families in a sensitive manner. The families referred to the researchers where the child had recovered from cancer were considered by the clinicians to be coping well. The ability of families to cope when the child is still receiving treatment was less apparent. The clinicians were understandably more anxious about involving these families in the study.

The consultant initially wrote to families to ask if they would be interested in taking part. The names of those that responded positively were given to the research team. A letter was then sent to each patient, all of whom were over 16 years of age. This was followed up with a telephone call to arrange an interview. At the end of the interview the patients were asked if they thought anyone else in their family had been affected by their illness. Their permission was then asked to approach other family members.

After the successful completion of the retrospective stage of the study the consultant was happy to allow families where the child was still receiving treatment or had recently finished to be approached. Again the consultant initially contacted families and gave the names of those who were interested to the research team. With this group the parents were contacted first and interviewed.

With their agreement, the patient and siblings, who were mainly under 16, were interviewed by the director of the project.

Finally, after the families in both groups had been interviewed, data was collected from the health professionals. The GPs in the prospective group were approached directly. Hospital staff were contacted after negotiation with their managers. The consultant expressed concern about interviewing the registrars, as at that point in time they were under a lot of pressure. However they were all happy to be interviewed.

Method of data collection

Semi-structured interviews were used to collect the data. The interview structure was based upon a model of assessment developed by Maguire and Faulkner (1988) which focuses on a respondent-led agenda. The optimum length of interview was 20–30 minutes and allowed time for key areas to be covered which the respondent may not have mentioned, but which were of importance.

The use of this approach proved very successful. Patients and their families were able to discuss their experiences, and know that the interviewee had listened. A typical comment was:

> It 'elps 'y you, you know, you talk same as 'ow this 'as 'elped me today . . . to talk about it . . . if you can't talk it hurts more.

The interviews were tape recorded with the respondent's consent for later transcription and analysis. Field notes were taken after the interviews, and comments made when the tape had been turned off were recorded if appropriate. Confidentiality was assured by assigning a number to each tape and transcript. The correlating list of names was kept separately in a locked filing cabinet.

The advantage of tape recording the interviews was that it made it easier to focus on what was being said. Tape recordings provide a detailed account of the interview yet such a wealth of information is often difficult to analyse and expensive to transcribe. Due to the emotive content of many of the interviews the impact on secretarial staff needed to be considered. The friendly and informal nature of the research centre meant that there was an awareness of how the secretaries felt about the content of tapes and formal support could be provided. However in different settings it may be necessary to provide a more informal approach to supporting secretarial staff. The team also needed to be aware of their support needs. Again this was provided on an informal basis.

Analysis of the data

Two complementary approaches, based upon Grounded Theory (Glazer and Strauss, 1967) were used to analyse the data. Families were placed in categories according to the degree to which they were 'coping' with the impact of childhood cancer, and themes that emerged from the data were examined.

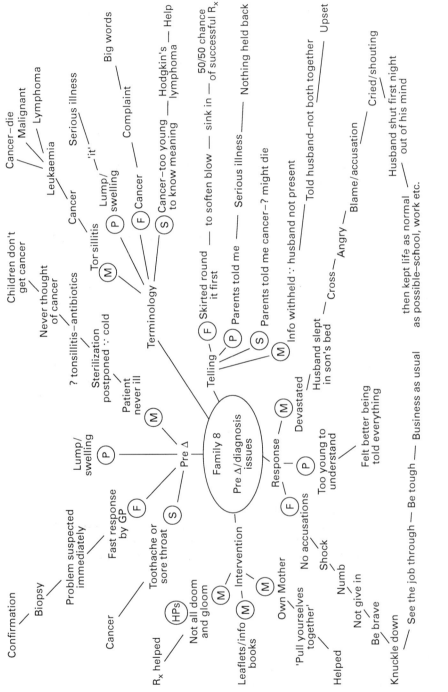

Figure 2.1 Example of a mind map; F = father; M = mother; P = patient; S = sibling; HP = health professional.

The use of categories of coping arose whilst undertaking the field work. The researchers became aware that families varied in the degree to which they 'coped' as a unit. Families were asked to define coping in their own situation and tell the researchers whether or not they were dealing with life as effectively as before diagnosis. Those who appeared not to be coping said that they could not function properly now as a result of changes in their lives caused by the cancer and its effect on family life. Families fell into one of three broad categories.

- **Category 1**   appeared to be in balance and coping without intervention.
- **Category 2**   reported problems at the time of illness and/or currently, with which they were coping but intervention could have been appropriate.
- **Category 3**   reported problems at the time of illness and/or currently, but did not appear to be coping.

The second level of data analysis involved examining themes that emerged from the data. The transcripts were studied in depth so that themes could be identified. Familiarity with the data enabled the researchers to identify themes. Analysis of this nature is time consuming and laborious. To enable maximum benefit from this work an approach known as 'mind mapping' developed by Buzan (1974) was used. Mind mapping works on the basis that the human brain does not function in a neat, linear fashion, and has limited concentration spans. In fact, the brain is able to work with many different ideas in a short space of time. At first sight such thought processes may appear unrelated. Mind mapping acknowledges this. To apply mind mapping the main theme or concept is written in the centre of a page. Other ideas which relate to it, even loosely, are noted and connected to the central theme with a line (see example of mind map – Figure 2.1). Recording themes and related ideas in this way enables the breadth and complexity of issues to be 'seen' more clearly.

CONCLUSION

The following chapters elaborate upon the results of the project. The breadth and sensitivity of the findings are evidence of the effectiveness of the methodology used. Facing the ethical dilemmas posed with a positive, open attitude provides valuable insight and suggests that this approach can be of use in similar settings.

REFERENCES

Bowling, A. (1992) *Measuring Health: A Review of Quality of Life Measurement Scales.* Open University Press, Milton Keynes.
Buzan, T. (1974) *Use Your Head.* BBC Publications, London.

Eiser, C. (1993) *Growing up with a Chronic Illness: The Impact on Children and their Families*. Jessica Kingsley Publishers, London.

Glazer, B.G. and Strauss, A.L. (1967) *The Discovery of Grounded Theory*. Weidenfield and Nicolson, New York.

Maguire, P. and Faulkner, A. (1988) How to improve counselling skills of doctors and nurses in cancer care. *British Medical Journal*, **297**, 847–9.

Melia, K. (1983) Student's views of nursing: discussion of methods. *Nursing Times*, **79**(20), 24–5.

Peace, G. (1994) Sensitive choices. *Nursing Times*, **90**(8), 35–6.

Shiva, V. (1989) *Staying Alive: Women, Ecology and Development*. Zed Books, London.

Sieber, K. (1992) *Ethically Responsible Research: A Guide for Students and Internal Review Boards*. Sage, London.

World Health Organization (1978) *Alma Ata – Primary Health Care; Health for All*. Series No 1. WHO, Geneva.

The Meaning of Cancer

3

You're just trying to pick on something what you can put your finger on
what's caused it, why has it come to him. All those rogues about, and
things like that, you're just searching for something to put your finger on
as to what it is.

Many people who hear they have cancer question what might have caused it
and ask, 'Why me?' When it is a child who is diagnosed it seems particularly
cruel. The irrational explanations for suffering and illness which often originate
in the more primitive layers of the psyche are brought into sharp relief as the
struggle ensues to make sense of what is happening and give shape and meaning to the chaos that threatens to overwhelm. A mother literally gave form to
her vision of what was happening to her family:

If he died . . . if he'd suffered, I'd feel kind of relieved that he wasn't
suffering anymore, but at the same time I would feel as though something
had been took away from me, it'd feel as though somebody may as well
chop a limb off . . . I mean I've always described meself, because I'm on
me own and I've got four children, I'm like a table with four legs and
take one leg away and I'd topple.

In this vivid analogy there is an agent – 'something', 'somebody' threatening to
strike at her and her family. For some the agent was a wrathful God dispensing
punishment to those who had sinned – but why a child as victim? One grandparent, shocked to see so many children and babies in a cancer ward said
'Why? They haven't done owt wrong?' Others, particularly parents, questioned
whether the cause was closer to home. Was it something they had done or not
done – fed their child with junk food, exposed them to a microwave, or stress
and anxiety over a messy divorce? Whatever the imagined cause, few parents
were able to escape feelings of guilt that in some way they had failed to protect
or nurture their child as they should. What was hard for most respondents to
accept was that the cause of childhood cancer might be more arbitrary and
random than this. A world with no apparent cause and effect, no pattern or

pattern-maker, seemed too frightening and uncertain a place to inhabit. Several respondents spoke of not knowing what was round the corner, the usual routine of their lives had been turned upside-down, now anything could happen, things were out of control and they felt helpless, even paralysed.

In this chapter some of the ways in which people made sense of the experience of childhood cancer are explored through an examination firstly of aspects of life before the diagnosis which appeared to influence how they responded to the diagnosis of cancer and secondly of the terminology used to describe the child's illness and the meaning they ascribed to it.

SIGNIFICANT EXPERIENCES BEFORE DIAGNOSIS

Earlier experiences, whether related to cancer or not, appeared to shape responses to the diagnosis.

Previous experience of cancer

Many respondents had some experience of relatives or friends who had cancer. For some this made things worse because the outcome was death, for others better. A sibling whose grandmother had died of cancer said it was upsetting watching her die but not **that** upsetting because she had wanted to die at the end and it was expected. This experience was, in a sense, measured against her brother's diagnosis of cancer, which was more upsetting because he did not want to die and it was unexpected. A grandmother, who had nursed her husband with cancer until his death, found it easier to understand her granddaughter's illness especially concerning the possibilities of treatment and how to take things day by day.

Three respondents from different families, a father and two grandmothers, said they had no previous experience of cancer. This seemed to add to their sense of disbelief and horror. The father on hearing the diagnosis of his daughter's brain tumour, wanted evidence such as an x-ray, but was too shocked to ask. The most difficult time for him was signing consent for the operation to go ahead, because he barely believed intervention was necessary.

Other significant experiences

Respondents from seven families recounted experiences in the past that did not concern cancer, but were, they felt, in some way related to the current experience of cancer. For most of them their child's diagnosis was seen as one of a series of traumatic experiences, the pain escalating with each experience with a sense of being overwhelmed should one more catastrophe occur. A mother told how her first child had died at birth from brain damage. Soon after her second child was diagnosed with cancer, it was discovered that her third had been severely deaf, probably from birth. For her, the series of traumatic experiences meant that she was a failure as a mother for not noticing her third child's deafness and subsequent difficulties in communication due to her attention being diverted to her child with cancer, and a failure at producing children. These feelings of guilt and inadequacy were despite the fact that she was also supporting a sick husband and was the main breadwinner in the family.

THE SEARCH FOR A CAUSE – SUPERNATURAL INTERVENTION

Several of these families, in recounting past experiences, seemed to be seeking a causative link. One father believed that the misfortune that had struck his family was his fault. Their first baby died with spina bifida, and their teenage child currently in remission, had had cancer as a baby. His father had also died of cancer. He believed all these tragedies were a punishment from God because he killed a man in active service. When he heard his daughter had cancer again he thought:

> Why are they picking on me again . . . I had to do national service – use my weapon . . . it's God paying me back for what I had to do . . . they're at me again . . . I feel guilty . . . the train robbers got off lighter than what I have . . . they got 30 years in prison, I've got the rest of my life.

This respondent was clinically depressed and had suicidal thoughts at the time of interview. He said:

> I just feel like going down the road and throwing myself on the railway lines, I'll be honest with you . . . I've thought if he takes me, he'll leave them alone.

This sense of a supernatural influence on the course of events, particularly the notion of 'a life for a life' was not uncommon. In one family the mother had had a miscarriage between her two eldest children. The patient, the third child, was an unplanned pregnancy described as 'a surprise package' and thought of as a replacement for the miscarriage. When later she was diagnosed as having cancer the mother said 'I thought it meant we weren't meant to have her'. Another mother said that just before her son was diagnosed she had been booked into hospital for sterilization, but she had a cold and the doctor postponed it. When she was told her son had cancer she felt terrible guilt:

> I couldn't comprehend why something that bad should happen to us as a family . . . was it something I'd done . . . went through the stage of feeling that because I'd gone to be sterilized it was God that had done this to [us].

For one family which was remarkable for its openness in communication, however, the course of events had a more fruitful explanation. They clearly believed, manifested in each family member's account, in the existence of some supernatural plan of events (God was not mentioned). The mother speaks for them, although the father, grandmother, eldest child Danny (who was the patient) and his sister, all told the same story in their own words. The mother was about three months pregnant at the time of her child's diagnosis. During the subsequent stressful weeks she miscarried:

> The day before [the miscarriage] I said to me mum 'if I've got to choose between Danny and this baby that I'm carrying I'd rather keep Danny . . . because I don't know this baby'. The day after I lost it . . . so, in a way it were like a sign to say well, you've got your way, Danny is gonna live. I'm glad it 'appened the way it did because erm, if it meant me carryin' 't baby through, then we mighta lost Danny. Things worked out okay.

When interviewed she had conceived and given birth to a third child which the 9 year old sister triumphantly explained was a replacement of the one mummy lost when Danny was ill. This family was possibly the poorest amongst all those participating, having no phone or car at the time their child was diagnosed and living in a deprived area. Yet they were also arguably the most cohesive and 'in balance'. It is possible that their belief that a pattern inheres in all life events helped them make sense of what was happening and gave their experience meaning and purpose.

TERMINOLOGY

The term 'cancer' was used by the majority of adult respondents. Some knew the correct name for the type of cancer but of these most did not know, before it was explained to them, that it was a form of cancer. An exception to this was the term 'leukaemia', which was recognized as a form of cancer – 'like on the telly, heard a lot about it'. The television was mentioned several times as a source of information about cancer, avidly watched for any applications to their own experience.

Interestingly a father of the one family who had prior knowledge of the correct terminology for his son's illness, Hodgkins disease, kept referring to 'the real nasties' when the diagnosis was in question, as if he couldn't bring himself to say the word 'cancer'. The fact that neither of his young sons mentioned the term cancer, although the father said they both knew that the illness was a form of cancer and its implications, suggests that there was a family trend to avoid the word. Other terms used included lump, tumour, mass, cancerous matter, and malignant, meaning 'it could spread', or 'grow' or 'come back'. With the exception of some children and teenagers these terms were used in the knowledge that the final diagnosis was cancer.

Meaning of terminology – children

Generally older children (9–14 years) realized that cancer was serious and life-threatening:

> . . . first thing I thought is was I going to die, because most things about cancer – people die over it.

But their fear of death was not always generated by what they had heard or from previous experience. Two patients were given the correct diagnostic label for their tumour and proceeded to look it up in a medical dictionary – as one explained 'because I weren't sure what it were'. It seems children can be very resourceful when they want to find out what is happening to them and adults are either protecting them or are unable to furnish them with the truth.

Younger children (7–9 years) who used the word 'cancer' were uncertain about its meaning, tending to relate it to the visible effects of treatment:

> When you have cancer all your hair falls out.

> . . . [the meaning of cancer is] about loss of 'air and treatment and injections.

An 8 year old patient said his mum had told him he had cancer on his left kidney. When asked what this meant to him he sounded disappointed:

> I thought it was original and when I found out, when I grew up, it weren't original.

He clearly enjoyed the rarity value and the ensuing attention it attracted!

Meaning of terminology – adults

The meaning of cancer for the majority of adult respondents was death. These are typical comments: 'death sentence', 'we thought it was t' end of everything', 'no-one's going to survive it', '[it means] a short time to live'. Some people thought of cancer as one illness and because of previous experience believed it spelt death. A mother said:

> I've lost me dad with that – God I'd got her in a coffin.

The power of the word 'cancer'

For some the word 'cancer' itself had malevolent power, evoking thoughts of death despite reassurances concerning possibilities of treatment. A grandmother said:

> I don't think that once that word were mentioned . . . I didn't cope at all. I'm not coping now. No I'm not.

She appeared to be obsessed with the word cancer and its negative connotations, unable to see anything positive in the experience despite her granddaughter's good progress and current state of remission. The majority, however, learnt that cancer did not automatically mean death and were able to adjust their view of it as a killer disease. A mother put the fear of 'the word' into perspective. Her own terminology and inadvertent use of clichés (in bold), are interesting and particularly apt in their meaning:

> a friend lives down the road, I mean she's **frightened to death** of the word cancer . . . but you've got to **learn to live with it** . . . you can't go to pieces because of the word cancer, it's just a word.

Another grandmother tried hard to rationalize her feelings, but her comment shows that once the word cancer had been used the sense of uncertainty prevailed:

> Cancer has always been a bad word in my thoughts . . . a lot of people you hear have died of it, it's a bit scary at first, whereas now we know that it can be combatted with treatment . . . but you're never sure.

ASPECTS OF DISBELIEF

Three aspects which were associated with the meaning of cancer appeared to contribute to some adults' initial disbelief of the diagnosis. Firstly many respondents commented on the youth of the patient – 'he's too young', 'he's had no life', 'why a bairn . . . you just think of cancer in old people. You don't realise young people get it'. There is a sense of unfairness, injustice, and also ignorance that cancer does not only afflict adults.

Secondly it was hard for some to relate cancer to a child who had been healthy before the diagnosis. A father said:

> It were a stunning blow . . . it made me feel a touch numb to think that the little lass who'd been running about basically the day previous, er, didn't look as if she'd got much longer with us.

And a respondent who took a long time to believe the diagnosis said:

> I couldn't believe it because to us he'd been running round and he'd been so full of life so . . . I couldn't understand how he could of suddenly got it.

Again the terminology used is poignantly apt: 'full of life'. Once the diagnosis had sunk in did this grandmother see her grandson as full of death?

Thirdly, in the aftermath of being told the diagnosis, some people could not believe this was happening to them: 'not my son . . . he's only 7 years old, it can't be right', 'she couldn't have it, somebody so close', 'I just thought it wouldn't happen to our family (this respondent was a nurse) she's so young . . . it's so rare'. Several spoke of feeling as though they were in a terrible dream world and would wake to find their child healthy and life back to normal.

But, despite these initial reactions of denial, it was a reality that eventually they all had to face. It was not uncommon, however, for parents and grand-parents to say that they wished they could redress the balance of nature which seemed to have got things the wrong way round, and take the place of their child or grandchild and bear the suffering themselves. It would make more sense – 'Why can't it be me? I've 'ad my life, she's all we've got'.

DISCUSSION

The search into past experiences that might in some way have caused the illness is clearly a painful one. Sadly there can be no adequate answers to these heart-felt questions. It is surely important, however, for professional carers to be aware of the influences that give meaning to this experience, for despite assur-ances given to families that it is not their fault that their child has cancer, there is evidence that some people find it ultimately hard to accept and are left with residual guilt.

An assessment of the family which includes an exploration of previous expe-riences which might have influenced their understanding of the current situation and appropriate explanation and support in the context of that understanding could help pre-empt denial and alleviate guilt. It seems that the points to be stressed are that there are different types of cancer, that the types, causes, effects and prognoses are different to adult cancers. And finally, whatever explanation and information is given, it is clear that the power of the word 'cancer' to evoke fears of recurrence and death cannot be overestimated.

The meaning that each individual gives to the experience of childhood cancer is multifaceted, dynamic and shaped by culture, experience and knowledge. Helping people to make sense of a situation which appears senseless and find meaning in what appears meaningless can make the difference between a posi-tive and negative experience, between hope and hopelessness and the courage to live through it and grow, or give up.

<table>
<tr><td>

4

</td><td>

The Patients

</td></tr>
</table>

Those who have cancer, be they adults or children, usually have a very clear memory of when they first realized that they were ill. Friends and relatives usually try to be protective at the point of diagnosis and this is particularly true of children. In this study children showed an acute ability to make sense of what was going on around them.

AF Can you remember how you first knew that you were ill?

P Well when I were in to General in Barnsley at first me mam and dad came in and I weren't allowed off t' bed and I weren't allowed to walk.

AF So you were taken into hospital and put into bed and told to stay there. What happened to get you into hospital?

P Well I had a bad nosebleed in t'early hours of morning and it went on for about half an hour and I just couldn't stop it so me mam phoned for an ambulance and they took me to hospital, had me in hospital, and then came back home and a couple of minutes after it started coming through t'pack and I had to go back again.

AF So you were perfectly well and you suddenly had this nosebleed. How did that feel?

P Scary . . . well when I went in they took a blood test and didn't say owt. They just like left me in t'room on me own and the doctor that took blood test took me mam and dad outside.

AF So you were left there not really knowing what was going on.

P Yeah that scared me as well.

This child was one of six boys in the prospective group and had been diagnosed with his cancer a year earlier. He was still frustrated at how little he had been told at the time that he had his first massive nosebleed. This clear memory and frustration was shared by those in the retrospective group as well. One teenager when asked if he remembered what he knew at the time said it was frightening, 'I knew it were like a growth of some kind, I asked for a dictionary and then I worked it out'. He was not happy that the information he needed was not readily available to him, but sensed that others were trying to protect him.

EFFECT ON NORMAL LIFE

Children in both the prospective and retrospective group were asked to describe the effects of their diagnosis on their normal lives (see Tables 4.1 and 4.2).

Table 4.1   Patients in the study

	Prospective	Retrospective	Total
Male	6	7	13
Female	3	2	5

Table 4.2   Effect on normal life

	Positive	Negative
Prospective	3	9
Retrospective	8	47

Surprisingly, most patients had some positive things to say about having a diagnosis of cancer. Not having to go to school was a plus for one of the children in the prospective group though this inability to lead a normal life through school and allied activities was seen as a negative by most children in the study. Most positive comments however were linked with the secondary gains of having a life-threatening disease. These included prayers at school and feeling special because of that, collections for presents that otherwise would not have occurred and the extra fuss and attention from the family. Interestingly the retrospective group remembered more positive aspects of finding that they had cancer than did the prospective group where only three positive comments were made. One of these was from a child who obviously found the hospital experience quite stimulating.

AF   So they took your lump out, but what was it like being in hospital?
P   Nice.
AF   It was nice, what did you like?
P   The food and cinema, they had a cinema there with a load of videos and we kept on watching the videos, they had games.
AF   So you had good food and games and videos to watch, so it was fun. Do you remember if you felt ill?
P   No.
AF   So you just had a good time. What about the other children there?
P   I made friends with one and in t'night we kept talking to each other when everyone else was asleep.

This child was seven when he was admitted to hospital.

The same hospital looked very different to a little girl who was admitted when she was ten.

AF   How did you like it in hospital?

P   Well it wasn't too good I didn't like the food and I kept feeling sick and I just felt awful. I didn't like it.

AF   So you felt too poorly to make friends or anything like that?

P   Well I made friends yeah, but I were alright at one moment and the next I felt poorly.

AF   So it really was a rotten time?

P   Yeah.

It can be seen that the child who didn't feel ill while in hospital could enjoy all the benefits of a new environment and stimulation while the child who did feel ill was more concerned by those feelings of illness than by what was going on around her. Another negative aspect added by a child who was six when she was admitted, was her belief that the nurses ordered her about, telling her to do this, that and the other.

It was interesting to look at the two groups of patients in terms of those negative comments, some of which were about the way that the hospital admission went but others that were to do with the restrictions that illness imposed on the children such as their ability to play, to be involved in things that were going on in their own locality, and their perceived loss of friends. In the prospective group there were nine negative comments some to do with the hospital but others to do with the impact of feeling different.

It could be argued that the retrospective group who were all in good remission would remember the more positive aspects of having been ill and the secondary gains that it brought. However, although their positive comments were more than those of the prospective groups their negative comments were considerably more, 47 negative comments being made. These comments covered the same areas as those of the prospective group but they seem to be remembered with more force and with some bitterness.

The fact that the retrospective group were all young adults had obviously given them time to add to their concerns. For example, one patient in the retrospective group saw a negative in terms of his hair not growing as thickly since chemotherapy and this fuelled his resultant belief that he would not ever marry though he really wanted to. He felt that all girls would find him unattractive.

Relationships

Perhaps the largest concern for both groups was the effect of their cancer on relationships, particularly within the family. When the effect on relationships was seen to be negative there were strong feelings of guilt, particularly in the patients. One for example, in the retrospective group, felt that her parents' marriage split-up was somehow due to her own illness where in fact the relationship had been rocky for some time. The child's illness may have been the final straw if it was responsible at all. Another child in the retrospective group was very worried about the effect of her illness on family members and as a result suffered panic attacks.

In the prospective group one child thought that his mother's miscarriage, just after he became ill, was his fault and directly related to the fact that he was ill. This belief was shared with his sister as was the resultant belief that their mother's subsequent pregnancy and successful delivery of a baby signalled the fact that the child with cancer was getting better.

The effect of the guilt engendered by the patients, taking responsibility for disruptions in relationships, led to a very clear role reversal where children in the study, from the very youngest at seven, felt that they had to keep their feelings from their parents in order to protect them. It will be seen that the siblings (Chapter 5) also had some role reversal in feeling that they had to protect the patients. The reactions and beliefs of one patient, aged seven and a half years, are shown in the following field notes.

Field Notes

P was looking out of the window for my arrival, greeted me with her mother and introduced the dog, took me to her bedroom, showed me Minnie Mouse – a present from Disneyland. I told her I had a Tigger and she then found a book about Pooh and read some of it. She then agreed to answer some questions and have the tape recorder on. After the tape recorder was switched off the following exchange took place.

AF	Thank you again for telling me about your illness.
P	It's alright.
AF	Do you talk to others like you've talked to me?
P	Shakes head.
AF	Mummy?
P	No.
AF	Why is that?
P	It would worry her, I mustn't make her sad.
AF	You think it still would?
P	Yes.
AF	Alright, shall we go down now?

Relationships with friends were also mentioned when children talked about the effect of their cancer on normal life. This mainly came after treatment had started and the first flush of good wishes and presents had stopped. Children were teased and called 'baldy', one was upset because the teacher would not initially allow her to wear a hat in school and most children felt that they were not well supported by adults when other children teased them. It says a great deal for the children's resilience that they were able to work through these problems and restore friendships that had been severed during their illness.

The overall impression from the children in the study, on their knowledge of the effect on relationships, showed considerable insight into the difficulties faced by others. In the retrospective group there was a particular awareness of the difficulties faced by their siblings. They were very aware that the siblings were getting less attention from family members and that this could affect the patient's relationship with his or her brothers and/or sisters. Here again guilt stepped in as the patients felt that they were being favoured because they were ill.

This awareness of family dynamics extended to grandparents, although one patient reported feeling closer to her grandparents as a result of the illness. In another family, relationships with the grandparents worsened and remained poor. This could have been because the grandparents tried to take over and organize parents but, from the patient's point of view, he felt wholly responsible for the fact that relationships were worse after he had become ill.

With the exception of the change in relationships at school and with friends where the patients felt that there was a lack of understanding beyond their control, the children appeared to take responsibility for the effects of their illness and therefore they took full responsibility for any adverse changes in family relationships.

ADJUSTMENT BACK TO NORMAL LIFE

When asked of the difficulties and pleasures in adjusting back to normal life there were both positive and negative responses. The prospective group felt much more positive about adjusting to home life unlike the retrospective group who continued to feel much more negative (Table 4.3). It could be argued that for the prospective group the joy of coming home was fresher in their minds but this also suggests, sadly, that the retrospective group have less pleasant memories given that only seven made positive comments about adjustment as opposed to 16 positive comments in the prospective group.

Table 4.3 Adjustments to normal life

	Positive	Negative
Prospective	16	8
Retrospective	7	38

The positive effects of adjusting back to normal life were largely to do with coming home.

AF How were things at home after you'd had the treatment and you were home again?

P I like had all me friends coming round and I didn't mind that cause we'd have a laugh and I'd ask them what happened at school, that wasn't so bad and everybody were buying me things and that.

These positive feelings were shared by other children in the study.

I liked it coming home cause everybody's kind to you. I kind of liked it cause I could get away with owt, I still like it now. I take everything as a joke.

The positive aspects of coming home were, for many children, tempered with the problems of returning to school.

AF How hard was it to get back into the swing of things?

P I didn't like going back to school at first cause I sort of felt like misplaced sort of thing, and one of the teachers he saw me wearing a hat and he come in and started shouting – but he didn't realize who I was and one of the teachers actually made a joke about me so I had to tell the head of the year.

AF Who did you tell?

P Head of the year, Mr Lee, cause he felt he were helping. If I wanted to come to school he'd come and fetch me and if I didn't feel well then he'd bring me home.

Another area linked with school that caused concern for some children was catching up on their work, especially if exams were looming. Again there were positives mixed with the negative aspects of catching up. One patient described how she had difficulty with her handwriting and how the school had provided her with a typewriter to ease the problem.

The negative comments from the retrospective group again covered similar areas to the prospective group though one child talked about how he felt that God couldn't love him anymore if he'd given him cancer. Memories of returning to school were also very strong in the retrospective group, one child described having to do a year again and being worried about getting to know people and making new friends. One child in the retrospective group described having to give up playing football until the treatment was finished. Another said:

> I had a bit of stick from the others [pupils], I got chased round the school for my hat when I first went so I used to escape that and the teachers had a word with the older years, I didn't want to go back the first time.

Overall the prospective group viewed their adjustment back to normal life in very positive terms and with few negative comments whereas the retrospective group saw very little that was positive in their adjustment to life with cancer. Only seven positive remarks were made against 38 negative comments. Again, the strength of the negative feelings is striking in the retrospective group even though it was obvious for the whole sample that considerable effort had been put in, by those around them, to help them to adjust to a normal life.

One child was so positive about his mother's efforts on his behalf that he had nominated her for a local award, of a bunch of flowers, and had been very thrilled when his nomination had been accepted. His mother described his gesture with tears in her eyes.

This is in sharp contrast to a male sibling who said that his sister who had had a brain tumour could never return to a normal life because he felt that her parents were treating her in such a special way that she would be changed for good. He saw these changes to be working in a negative way. This comment was about his sister who had become very quiet and withdrawn after coming home from hospital. He was obviously quite concerned about her facial paralysis.

CHANGES IN LIFE DURING REMISSION

Most patients reported some change in themselves during remission as a result of having had cancer and treatment. In this area of questioning there were fewer differences in positive and negative aspects of change. In the prospective group for example there were four positive comments and four negatives. In the retrospective group there were 10 positive comments and 14 negatives (Table 4.4). In the prospective group the equal number of positive and negative factors of change suggest that there is some sense of balance which is evident in the following comment:

> Before I started treatment I was sort of, I had serious side and I'd mess about when you could mess about but I'd be serious when I had to. And when I were on treatment I were a quiet sort of person then. On last course of treatment, when I had cancer, I thought – well – what am I getting worried for? I'll have to finish the course or I'm going to die

anyway so what does it matter so I just take life as a joke, and I don't get bothered about it now.

Table 4.4   Changes in remission

	Positive	Negative
Prospective	4	4
Retrospective	10	14

This quiet balance from a 14 year old lad did have its more serious side which came out when he was asked how he viewed his future. 'Like now I feel fine but if I bang myself I think well it might be cancer again.' Some children felt that they had improved in certain areas as a result of their illness – one child described how poor he was at playing football before his treatment, and how he improved dramatically when he came back. He put this down to his chemotherapy.

This feeling that the cancer might return was a feature of both the prospective and retrospective group. This is particularly surprising in the retrospective group where all patients were in very good remission yet almost all reported some level of fear that their cancer might return. Many described treating every bump, bruise or headache as a potential sign that their illness was returning and one of the retrospective group said 'I try not to think a lot really because I find it depressing'.

There was a positive side to the realization that life expectancy could not be taken for granted, particularly in the retrospective group. One patient said, 'it made me feel that you can't take owt for granted, people think, oh I'm living but you can't take life for granted and I found that out at the age of ten'. This same patient later said 'I'm more careful and cautious about life now I accept the value of life more now about thinking what it is, because you think to your-self it's only life. They don't realize how quickly it can be took away from you. It can be took just like that. They don't realize that but I make the most of it.'

This feeling that there is a need to make the most of life was taken to the extreme by a lad who having recovered from cancer was currently suffering from Perthes disease, possibly acquired as a result of radiotherapy. He was registered disabled and awaiting a hip replacement. When asked how he saw his future he said he wanted to be a stand-up comic and he might be a millionaire one day. He would then buy me a drink if I came to watch him perform.

Many patients reported an added toughness that had not been there before the illness. This toughness led some of the patients, particularly in the retrospective group, to be able to joke about their disablement. One of the girls in the retro-spective group had had an arm amputation. She reported sunbathing topless on holiday in Spain and made a joke about her false arm slipping when a new boyfriend tried to give her a cuddle. Another 12 year old girl was taunted at the local youth club by a boy who said, 'cancer freak, cancer freak, I've got more hairs round my willy than you've got on your head.' The patient responded 'Oh yes, let's see', and she and her cousin jumped on the lad and pulled his trousers off. This girl reported that she would not have been able to do anything as brave as that, or as naughty, before she was ill.

Life then changed for all patients in the sample. For some there was a raised awareness of the effect of their cancer on others, for some there was the beginnings of spiritual awareness and for most patients, the realization that life must be enjoyed today because tomorrow is uncertain. Perhaps the major change however, was an added 'toughness' emerging from handling a serious disease and an uncertain future.

ATTITUDE TO CHECK UPS

Attitudes to check ups among the patients were positive with no negative comments being made. For example:

AF   When you've been to the hospital to see the doctor do you want it to be any different?

P   No it's perfect the way it is.

AF   You sound as though you've been a very brave girl. You go to the hospital and it doesn't upset your life at all, that's great. So do you think you've told me all about it now?

P   Yes.

This response was typical of children talking about being followed up. They used such words as 'reassuring'. Some mentioned the fact that check ups were okay because there were not usually blood tests involved. One child said, 'I like the doctor because she tickles me.'

What is interesting here is that the only negative comments were made by mothers, one grandmother and two siblings – and those comments were all in the area of being reminded of the cancer with one sibling feeling that the patient going for a check up reminded him of all that his brother had been through.

LIVING WITH CANCER

It will have been seen in this chapter that although there are secondary gains of being ill in terms of presents, fuss and attention, most children in the study felt some negative responses of the trauma of having cancer and these negative responses, rather than going away, were amplified in the retrospective group particularly showing how their cancer was now an integral part of their lives even though they were in good remission.

There are some very important points, however, not least that many of the patients' negative responses and memories were concerned with their own emotional response to what was going on around them. This included guilt for feeling that unhappy life events must in some way be tied to their own illness, and this showed the underlining of responsibility in the child for having become ill.

This sense of guilt for having become ill was especially strong when family relationships had become more difficult after the illness, particularly if a marriage that was already in trouble had broken up.

One point that came through quite clearly in comparing the patients' attitudes to their cancer with those of other family members was that the patient on the whole felt quite well supported by those around them although some unhappy incidents took place such as teasing, this was soon cleared up once the situation became known and most patients felt very supported by letters and visits from school friends and teachers.

One area where children did feel there had been problems was in getting back to school and catching up. Only one patient had a home tutor to enable this catching up to happen and his sister felt that the tutor not only helped her brother to catch up but had also been the key to restoring the child's self-confidence. The last word must go to a young male patient who seemed to be in total balance about his cancer.

AF   If you could look back over the last year and change anything what would you change?

P   I don't know really, I suppose probably actually having cancer.

AF   So it sounds as if you would have liked not to have had it, but feel that the handling of it has been okay. Is that what you're saying?

P   Yeah. I'm not sure really.

AF   There's nothing that you can think, 'If that had been different I would have been happier'?

P   It'd probably have to be that, just not having it, but you don't really know what's going to happen in life in the future cause if I hadn't had it then I might have got it later on in life and the doctor said I have age and fitness on me side so that'd help me along, so what I'm really saying is sooner rather than later I think.

AF   Is there anything else you'd like to say about being ill?

P   Not really, no.

5

The Siblings

> I feel as though I'm Sam's sister and I'm not me. About four or five
> months ago I went to the shop up the lane and a woman came in and said
> 'How's your sister?' I said she was alright. 'That's alright then'. Then I
> just came home crying because I felt that's how everybody knew me.

This teenager, Chris, was interviewed five years after her sister had been diagnosed with cancer. Recalling the experience was particularly painful for her –
she cried gently as she spoke, yet was able to express her feelings in graphic
detail. She explained how she found it hard to remember her life before her
sister's illness but since the diagnosis every aspect was clear. She had thought
of running away from home, not because she couldn't get on with her sister and
parents, but because she felt unable to be herself, she had to suppress her iden-
tity. Instead of taking this step she had learnt to 'put a lining over myself so that
I won't get hurt'. Her real self sometimes emerged in school where she became
more assertive, but the lining was put back on as soon as she arrived home. Her
plan was to leave home when she was able to earn her own living and move to a
place where nobody knew about her background. Her ideas about her choice of
career were revealing. She said:

> I'd like to do something that will help other people where I can speak my
> opinion . . . and say what I'd like others to do . . . because I feel every-
> body's always told me what to do and so I feel like turning the tables
> round and me doing it for a change.

It could be argued that these are the words of the average teenager rebelling
against authority. While there may be an element of this the feelings Chris
expressed were common to many of the siblings interviewed in an age range
between seven and early twenties, although the younger age group (7–12) were
perhaps not so articulate. Also there was no evidence that her anger and frustration were directed at her parents who she described as warm and loving. She
couldn't tell them about her distress because she felt 'they had enough on their
plate with Sam's illness'. Her feelings were caused by the **situation** not figures

of authority as her ambivalent behaviour underlines – it cost her much effort to present one persona at home and another at school.

Although the sample of siblings was small (17 in total) this teenager's account of how her life was disrupted, her reactions to her sister's illness, and her subsequent changes in view on life are representative of the group. Furthermore the results of this study, which suggest that siblings suffer more than their ill brother or sister in terms of unattended emotional needs, are supported by previous research.

All siblings over 16 were approached individually to negotiate an interview, as were patients over 16. Parents were approached for permission to talk to those under 16. All were interviewed on their own with the assurance that what they said would not be passed on to any other member of the family without permission. This allowed free expression without threat. It was interesting to note that two of the siblings specifically asked to be interviewed, before being approached, as though anxious not to be left out and eager to give their side of the story. One did not want to be interviewed but agreed to fill in a questionnaire. There were also some omissions: For example, some had been too young at the time of diagnosis to remember what had happened and were not approached. There were five refusals. Of these one refused outright, three in one family voted with their feet and were not around at the time of interview – the mother explained they were too shy – and the mother of another family felt it would upset both her children, the patient and his brother, and refused access on their behalf.

Table 5.1 Siblings in the sample

	Siblings		
	Prospective	Retrospective	Total
Brothers	5	1	6
Sisters	4	7	11

To find out how the impact on each family member changed over time they were asked about how they felt during three stages of the illness: Firstly, after the diagnosis was made; secondly, during the period of adjustment to the diagnosis and whilst treatment was underway; and thirdly, after treatment had finished. The number of negative and positive comments for each stage were recorded (see Tables 5.2, 5.3 and 5.4). It is important to point out, however, that a high score (either negative or positive) does not relate to the intensity of feeling. A sibling with an acute memory of all the bad things that happened during that time might not be suffering as deeply as a sensitive, imaginative sibling, whose one fear was being left alone at home whilst the rest of the family was visiting hospital, preoccupied with fearful fantasies, far worse than reality, about what was happening.

EFFECT ON NORMAL LIFE

The term 'normal' is an ambiguous word in that it has a different meaning for different people. In this study its meaning derived from the perspective of each person interviewed. Siblings were asked about how their lives had changed from what they had been before their brother or sister had been diagnosed with cancer, how their feelings changed and how they coped with those changes over time. The changes were measured against what had been their usual or 'normal' pattern of life.

Table 5.2   Effect on normal life

		Positive	Negative
Siblings	Prosp $N = 9$	3	16
	Retro $N = 8$	8	24
Total		17	11	40

Possibly the biggest change for siblings was that they received far less attention from their parents; some were looked after by relatives or friends which could entail being away from home. Feelings were mixed. Mostly they missed the contact – 'not knowing what were goin' off', but even the youngest realized that their ill brother or sister needed their parents more. This seems to be the source of the ambivalence Chris described so vividly. Siblings were very aware of the distress and subsequent effects on family relationships caused by such a crisis and were anxious not to add to the general upset of 'normal' family life – 'I had to be alright' one said; yet they were as frightened and bewildered as their parents but with less ability to find someone to trust with their fears and provide them with information. Some feared they might catch or inherit cancer; some felt guilty they might have caused or contributed to their brother or sister's illness. Their usual source of comfort and reassurance at difficult times, a parent, was either absent or preoccupied with the ill brother or sister. One teenager said:

> Everybody used to do things for him in the family and I like got pushed to one side. Well, they probably still thought of me, but wi' me being older, well she can look after herself and that.

The parents' preoccupation with the ill child had its positive side, however, for another teenage sibling, Phil, who spoke of the advantages of being left to his own devices:

> When they came home [from hospital] they didn't have much time for me, but it didn't bother me . . . I was 16 nearly 17 and at that age you

resent everything they do . . . They didn't know that I didn't go to double chemistry on Tuesday afternoons – it was boring. I could get away with it.

Later in the interview Phil confessed that his brother's illness had probably affected him more than he'd realized. When asked if the family had talked about it and its implications when they were together, he said:

Not on a deep basis, just day to day things – nothing that he might die or anything . . . Things aren't talked about. I don't think it's just our family, it's how things are . . . it's just not done, it just doesn't happen. It's the same with my mate's Dad who committed suicide this Summer and it's never talked about there. Things aren't ever said.

So it seems that even if the family is not split by responsibilities of care and do have time together, such is the pain of confronting and sharing uncertainties and undisclosed feelings, parents may be absent in spirit if not in fact as far as the sibling is concerned.

While for some the lack of attention was compensated for by being spoilt by relatives, many siblings were anxious for more opportunities to talk to their parents, partly to tell them about how they were feeling and partly to have more information about what was going on and how their brother or sister was progressing. An aunt who was looking after her nephew some distance from the family home said he was nagging her to ring home all day to find out what was happening.

The other aspect of a sibling's life which was disrupted was school. However, apart from two teenagers who were approaching exams and found difficulty in concentrating – their thoughts on their ill brother or sister rather than school work – there was little comment about school until the brother or sister themself returned.

It does seem that initially the major area of problems for siblings stems from a lack of information and reassuring contact with a parent, someone who can give them immediate feedback about what is going on, provide accurate details and share the pain of assimilating the crisis that has hit them all, so that they can gradually become aware of and understand each others' fears and give mutual comfort in their distress.

ADJUSTMENT TO NORMAL LIFE

Siblings were, in the main, relieved to see their brother or sister back at home and beginning to pick up the threads of a disrupted routine:

He's playing football again . . . been getting good marks in his exams and that, so he's really caught up with things.

But what was clear, particularly in the prospective group all of whom were in the throes of adjusting, was that life for themselves was far from easy in comparison with their ill sibling.

Table 5.3   Adjustment to normal life

		Positive	Negative
Siblings	Prosp $N = 9$	2	13
	Retro $N = 8$	0	4
Total		17	2	17

Being out of hospital and back in familiar surroundings was understandably a positive factor for the ill child. Moreover they were still given preferential treatment by family and friends:

He gets his own way a lot more now – I still feel left out . . . Now he's not poorly he should be treated as normal.

Despite a lingering resentment at the extra attention given to the ill sibling, anxieties and fears about whether they were really getting better, and a subsequent protectiveness towards them appeared to predominate in siblings' responses. Sometimes these anxieties were fuelled by the all too visible side effects of treatment, such as baldness, loss of weight and weakness, which well siblings were not exposed to initially as much as parents since they did not usually visit the hospital as frequently. The patient's first arrival home seemed literally to bring home to them how ill their brother or sister had been. One patient on return home, bald and several stones lighter than he had been, was horrified to be greeted by his 4 year old brother with the exclamation 'Who's that monster?'

In older siblings, from 7 years, the reactions were more of protectiveness and wanting to look after their brother or sister both at home and defending them from bullying at school. But even this role was not easy. A 15 year old brother said about the period just after his sister's homecoming:

I just remember her being so ill when she was laying there all day. She wasn't the sister I knew. That made me feel bad . . . it was obviously difficult, she couldn't do certain things . . . so we had to do it for her and often . . . well she'd be lying there with a blanket over her and everything and you'd ask her if she wants anything and she'd go 'no', and you're not really sure whether she does or not so you keep asking her, and finally she says 'no, no'.

Several siblings experienced similar confusion in how to handle the situation. It demanded a different kind of relationship, almost as if they were having to get to know a different brother or sister – 'She wasn't the sister I knew'. Another 9 year old said, when his brother came out of hospital and he returned from staying with a relative, 'it took me a bit to get used to my brother after being in hospital and not being together'. The difficulty of getting back to normal relationships was compounded by his mum saying 'leave [your brother] alone, he's been ill don't you know'.

This behaviour of taking on a parental role, apparent even in 7 year olds, was particularly evident in sisters. One sister said that before her elder brother's diagnosis **he** had protected **her** but now roles were reversed and she 'mothered' him. There is a strong sense of having to grow up quickly and take on a new responsibility – a younger sister by two years said:

> I've got all this responsibility that I've got to take care of her doing things. . .'

and an older sister:

> I thought I might lose my little brother so I started to do everything I possibly could for him.

One sister who was 8 years old at the time of her 6 year old brother's diagnosis, was clearly deeply affected by him looking so ill. When interviewed nine years later, aged 17, she was in tears as she recalled the effects of the treatment, 'his hair falling out, the drips and everything'. Yet she also enjoyed the role of 'mollycoddling' him and remembered playing at nurses when she visited him in hospital, and protecting him from bullying when at school. Normally a passive child, she described how she had 'thumped' a boy two years older than herself for teasing her brother and got upset when she wasn't around to 'have a go' at his tormentors. She added:

> I feel very protective to him still . . . still really close. I used to worry about him all the time . . . but he's changed, he seems to want to be really strong and macho these days. Probably growing up . . . he doesn't like being mollycoddled.

When asked, 'How does that make you feel?' she began to cry again:

> I don't know – redundant . . . I just feel as though I should be looking after him all the time, but he doesn't want it. To look at him now you would never think there was anything wrong with him would you?

Clearly the initial disruption to 'normal' life can have long-term effects.

CHANGES IN LIFE DURING REMISSION

It is interesting to note that the positive and negative factors are evenly balanced overall at 16, although the retrospective group appear in the long term to view permanent changes as more negative than positive. It does seem, however, that there were many gains in terms of improved relationships. These are a few typical comments:

Table 5.4   Changes in remission

		Positive	Negative
Siblings	Prosp $N = 9$	8	3
	Retro $N = 8$	8	13
Total	17	16	16

She's become more special.

It's brought us closer – we used to fight like cat and dog. We still do but it brought us closer.

He's improved at school . . . gained in confidence . . . it's drawn us closer together . . . it's nice being with him because he seems more grown up – we'd do anything for each other now . . . I love to do things for him, 'cos I couldn't give him that when he was poorly . . . I can talk to him more than I can me own Mum and Dad.

Not only were there closer feelings between siblings. A brother said:

My relationship with Mum and Dad has sort of been closer . . . I can be in the room and my Mum and Dad can be discussing about what's happening to [the patient] . . . and they have't told [the patient] but they actually told me. Now before I used to be in the room and Mum says, 'can I just have a word with Dad' sort of . . . I feel a lot more adult. They treat me as being more grown up and they can discuss things more freely with me around.

This same 15 year old sibling went on to say that the family had always been 'homely, caring, helping and supporting' but had become 'even more supporting and understanding of each other'. Another simply explained the cohesiveness which helped them win through:

It were tough . . . but once your family helped you, you get there in the end.

Despite this spirit of optimism and the conviction of several younger siblings that their brother or sister was now well, concerns about the possibility of recurrence were voiced by some teenage siblings:

> I'm frightened in a way for if it ever comes back . . . you just can't forget it, it will always be there, thinking if it ever came back it would be worse.

> I just worry about it recurring . . . there's always that chance.

Similarly to parents and grandparents teenage siblings seemed to adopt a philosophical attitude reflecting a new maturity:

> I've come to realize you don't know when your number's up so you've got to live every day, not necessarily as your last one, but you've got to take all your opportunities. It's no use saying 'Oh I can go tomorrow'. If an opportunity comes to try something out or see something you've not seen, take it.

But this maturity was tinged with the bravado of youth:

> You might as well just blow it because you might not be here tomorrow and have a good time!

DISCUSSION

When the totals of positive and negative comments are looked at separately, the prospective and retrospective groups are different in relation to the ill sibling (the patient) and to the pattern of change over time. On the graph (see Fig 5.1) it can be seen that the 'retrospective' patients and siblings look back on the experience as most negative; they do not come out of the negative pole throughout the course of the illness. The patients recorded a greater number of negative comments than siblings, which is in contrast to the prospective group, though interestingly they coincide in their view of permanent changes to their lives. A reason for the greater number of negative comments made by the retrospective group may be that they were an older age group and more articulate or had not been given an opportunity to talk when going through the experience and when given a licence to do so embellished their memories with a teenage flourish – we all add colour to our past in this way and accepting that it happens should not imply that the strength of feeling or distress is any less than that recalled.

The difference in change over time between the 'prospective' patient and sibling is particularly interesting in its volatile nature. The healthy sibling

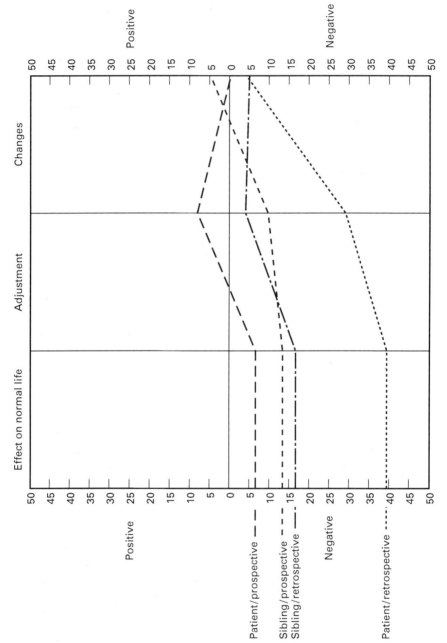

Figure 5.1 Positive and negative comments

starts lower in the negative pole than the patient, hardly lifting during adjustment, then rising quite steeply to look positively at the changes in his or her life – the only member of the family to do so on this scale. The explanation for the difference may be due to a factor emphasized in the literature, that children respond to the immediate rather than dwelling on the future. Siblings' lives are affected drastically when the patient is first diagnosed. Life is not easier during the first stages of adjustment because they are more involved with the day to day care, become more aware of how ill the patient has been and still feel pushed out – for the prospective siblings this is current experience, for the retrospective a bad memory, dulled by time. The 'prospective' sibling perhaps feels that the future can only improve if the ill brother or sister has recovered, hence the rise into the positive pole. The fact that the 'prospective' patient does not reflect the same optimism, or maintain the positive feelings experienced once treatment is over is perhaps because it is **they** who have gone through the life-threatening experience and, in a way which mirrors the reactions of the adult members of the family, the future has become a more definite concept than children who have not had this experience are able to apprehend, even if, ironically, a painfully uncertain one.

For the retrospective group, discussing permanent changes was about the immediate situation and, while things were not as bad as after the diagnosis, life (as in Chris's experience) had changed. These seemed to be unresolved issues which siblings, careful to conceal from parents at the time of crisis to protect them from further distress, were still struggling with. One sister said 'I used to just sit and cry and think about it and not be able to do anything'. As with Chris, her feelings persisted.

The severity and long term nature of the effects on siblings is documented in previous research, and intervention such as peer support groups has been evaluated with mainly positive results. Support groups on their own, however, although beneficial in sharing and expressing common fears and feelings, may not be enough to alleviate the problems of those siblings, such as some of those found in this study, where relationships and roles changed within the family. It seems that a family-orientated approach may be more appropriate in these circumstances.

Intervention designed to assess and strengthen family relationships without losing sight of each individual's distress is a skilful task, but not necessarily as great a strain on resources as it sounds. For example it could be helpful to counsel parents not to send healthy siblings away at the time of diagnosis if they can possibly manage to cope and to help them communicate more effectively and share the information they receive from specialists with all their children along with their inevitable distress.

Siblings live the longest with the impact that childhood cancer has on their lives. They experience the upheaval in family relationships at a critical time in their development. It seems of particular importance that their needs are assessed and attended to throughout the course of the disease and beyond, to help make the experience more positive and to harness the spirit, strength and energy for resilience, humour, and compassion so evident in the siblings who participated in this study.

The Parents | 6

Parenting is a demanding job which is generally learned through trial and error. When a child has cancer, parents enter a nightmare world where the terrain is unfamiliar, the future uncertain and their skills are challenged to the utmost. From the moment of diagnosis 'normal' life ceases and may never return to what it was before. A father said:

> I've seen some big events in my life, they all mean very little now . . . I'd never be able to put the experience of cancer at the back of me mind . . . I've a different outlook.

This chapter explores the impact of the diagnosis on parents, how life changed for them from diagnosis, through adjustment, to life beyond the illness. The experience was not all dark. For many there were positive aspects which helped to illuminate the way forward. These too are explored along with suggestions from parents which they felt might ease the experience. Chapter 10 addresses in more detail the ways in which families can be helped to **live** with cancer. The perspective of the father and the mother are mostly considered separately but in the context of relationships within the whole family.

To discover how the impact on parents changed over time, they were asked about how they felt during three stages of the illness: firstly, after hearing the diagnosis; secondly, during the period of adjustment to the diagnosis and whilst treatment was underway; and, thirdly, after treatment was finished. The number of negative and positive comments for each stage were recorded. This method not only allows for changes to be observed but also comparisons can be made between members of the family and between the prospective and retrospective groups of families. It is important to point out, however, that a high score (either positive or negative) does not relate to the intensity of feeling. For example a mother who had a score of five negatives in the treatment period and one negative in the period after treatment said the worst time for her was dealing with the fear of recurrence when treatment was over and she was back at home without the reassurance of the specialists and support of other families going through the same thing.

HISTORY OF PRESENT ILLNESS PRIOR TO DIAGNOSIS

The symptoms of cancer are often vague and slow to develop. They may be misdiagnosed as 'growing pains', 'school phobia' or appendicitis. Parents may have to take their child many times to the doctor and hospital for consultations and investigations before a final diagnosis is made. The way in which this stage of the child's illness is handled clearly influences how parents respond when they are faced by the person who confirms their worst fears.

Ten out of 19 parents had some complaint about health professionals at this time. These mainly related to late diagnosis. Three GPs were implicated. One was blamed for 'total negligence', another for 'misinterpretation of a biopsy' and a third who was 'slow to realise the significance of the symptoms'. In the case of the first two the family changed their GP. One is the subject of litigation – 'not because we want compensation but to make them realize the possible consequences of their mismanagement'.

The remainder were complaints about District General Hospitals. In one case the parents said the hospital lost their child's notes and they were generally 'messed about'. In another the parents were not told their child's appendix had been normal until months after an appendicectomy following a history of abdominal pain and constipation, when the patient returned for further investigation. A common complaint from mothers was that doctors would not listen to what they were saying about their children.

There was also the sense that the first doctor the parents saw with the presenting symptoms could have picked up the clues that this was a serious complaint but didn't. For example a parent said the first doctor wasn't 'a proper doctor', another said 'it wasn't our own doctor'. Another said that after returning to casualty several times seeing and being dismissed by the same doctor each time they finally saw a different one:

> 'She sussed it . . . she knew what she was doing . . . it weren't picked up when it should.'

These delays caused parents to feel anger and mistrust for health professionals and fear that the delay meant the disease had progressed to the stage that the child might not respond to treatment. Some also felt guilt. One mother couldn't bear to think back to the time before diagnosis because she felt so ashamed at forcing her child to go to school when she complained of feeling unwell. She believed this sense of guilt affected her current relationship with her child which tended towards over-protectiveness.

Not all comments about this stage were negative. A swollen tonsil was quickly recognized by a GP as potentially serious. The parents realized that some doctors would have passed it off as tonsillitis and were grateful for the speedy referral to the specialist. For another child the diagnosis was reached through an accident – a fall, resulting in a visit to casualty where a blood test revealed the necessity for further investigation. The fall was described as 'a Godsend'.

DIAGNOSIS

Telling the diagnosis

There is no way of softening the blow for parents when telling them their child has cancer. The experience can be made more harrowing and confusing, however, through inept handling both before and at the time of breaking the bad news. Parents who have gone through a number of misdiagnoses may not believe the doctor. A father, whose son's disease had progressed, undiagnosed, to the point of his imminent collapse, was very angry when he was finally told the diagnosis at the District General Hospital:

> I felt as if I was being condescended to – patronized.

The mother said:

> I didn't like him from the word go. He spoke to us as though we were ignoramuses . . . he thought I was just fussing . . . he started blinding us with science and gave the wrong information.

Anger is not uncommon however caringly a parent is told. One mother recalls:

> I remember swearing at 'im and saying 'you're lying to me' and trying to grab 'old of 'is neck.

But others have cause:

> I wanted to hit him . . . to think he could be so callous. That were my baby in bed an he just came and said she's got cancer.

This mother was told the diagnosis 'casually', in the corridor, without her husband present. This was unusual. Complaints of this nature invariably concerned staff at District General Hospitals. Typically the parents were told the diagnosis at the specialist children's hospital, by the consultant paediatric oncologist, together, in a consulting room, with a specialist nurse or social worker present. There was, in some cases, a sense of relief when parents came to the end of long drawn out investigations. A diagnosis, however frightening in its implications, meant that they knew what they were facing and they were in the best place to begin doing something about it. These are some of the aspects parents appreciated when they were told the news that was to change their lives:

They're so direct whatever is wrong they do tell you, they've got to tell you and I thought well I could put my faith in this lady.

(Mother)

She never ever gi' false 'ope . . . gave you the facts as they were.

(Mother)

Being listened to – that was a breath of fresh air.

(Father)

. . . efficiency . . . but relaxed atmosphere which meant that you felt as if you weren't imposing on them, that you had a right to be there and that they were going to do something.

(Father)

It was good to have it out in the open.

(Mother)

Effects of diagnosis

All families experienced shock on hearing that their child had cancer. This was expressed in various ways: 'stunned', 'devastated', 'I was in hysterics . . . just as though my world had come to an end', 'I went haywire'.

Some felt physically affected: 'It were like something hitting me . . . it were a physical feeling', 'I felt sick, I couldn't stop shaking', 'it's like a wave which comes over you . . . it's a funny sort of numb sensation'.

Several spoke of disbelief for various reasons: 'It didn't sink in', 'came out of the blue', 'couldn't be happening to us', 'we didn't trust the doctors', 'we were hoping they had got it wrong'.

Disbelief seems to be a form of coping by denial that this is happening after the immediate reaction of shock. It seems it is linked to a sense of helplessness and confusion. Parents said as the news began to sink in, 'I thought, how will I cope?', 'What can you do?'.

For many there then followed the difficult period of questioning 'Why me?', discussed in more detail in Chapter 3, when parents try to make sense of what is happening. The accompanying sense of turmoil this family feels is vividly illustrated:

What we done to deserve this? . . . you wonder what . . . 'ow it's happened . . . what 'ave we . . . is it summat we've done?

The line of questioning often leads to wondering about the cause of the cancer. Mothers in particular felt guilty that they might be to blame in some way for causing their child's illness. But the most extreme case was a father who believed **he** had brought the tragedy of his child's illness on the family. He thought it was a punishment from God because he had killed a man on active service.

With these feelings of shock, helplessness, confusion, questioning, blame and anger, it is not surprising that one of the major impacts on relationships between all family members, including friends and neighbours, was not wanting to communicate – wanting to 'block it out'.

> I couldn't do nothing. I just sat in the middle of the floor there in front of the fire and did nothing but look at the four walls . . . I didn't want anyone to come near me. I didn't want anyone to knock on t' door and I didn't want anyone to feel sorry for me. I just didn't want nobody.
>
> (Mother)

Some husbands and wives found difficulty in talking to each other. Fathers in particular found it difficult to talk about their feelings:

> I was always upset wi' it – I've always found it hard to talk about it. [Patient and wife] were more open than I were. I always got more upset.
>
> (Divorced father)

Two fathers admitted that they felt they should be strong in front of the rest of the family though they felt like crying. An interesting reflection on this gender difference is that more of the fathers in the retrospective group cried openly when recalling the experience of being told their child had cancer than those in the prospective group. This suggests that they had suppressed their grief over several years (from 2–11 years) through the child's treatment and recovery and were only able to give it expression when given 'permission' through the acceptable medium of a research interview.

One father appeared to have suppressed his feelings so successfully that he could not recall how he had accused his wife of being the cause of their child's illness, nor the fact that he had shut himself away the night after the diagnosis and would not share their sense of despair together. His wife remembered, but gently accepted that he wanted to deny what had happened – that it was his way of coping. They appeared to have achieved a degree of balance in their lives eight years after the diagnosis but their relationship seemed to be built on a brittle structure. The father frequently used metaphors of control: 'we had to knuckle under . . . be as tough as we could . . . get stuck in . . . tackle it head on . . . essential not to throw in the towel. . . it's not going to beat us, we're going to beat it', as though to wrench life into a pattern of his own making. Of his current relationship with his son he said:

> He doesn't cause any trouble really, just he's beginning to sort of flex his muscles and sometimes he gets a bit stroppy and I just have to remind him of the relative position in the family.

Should that control be threatened by some further trauma it is questionable whether the structure would hold.

This couple were not alone in what could be called a mismatch of perception between husband and wife. Another example was a husband who said he felt the relationship with his wife had become closer since the diagnosis. His wife, however, felt they had drifted apart because she had had to bear the brunt of hospital visiting as well as keep her job going as she was the breadwinner of the family due to her husband's chronic illness – they had had so little time to be together and talk – she had become used to running what the GP called 'a tight ship' on her own. These 'mismatches' underline the importance of assessing parents separately, indeed all members of the family where resources permit, as each experiences the same situation in a different way and do not necessarily communicate their feelings to those closest to them.

Another concern of parents was how they should communicate with their children:

> You think about how's he goin' to go on . . . you can't explain it, nobody's goin' to explain to 'im what it's like.

Parents were encouraged to be open with their children but they clearly had some difficulty with this, wanting to protect them. A father said:

> We do try and keep these sort of fears separate from the boys and jolly them along . . . not lying to them but just telling them the truth in a sort of easy way.

The parents of this family decided the patient's 10 year old sibling should be sent away to a close relative immediately after the diagnosis was made. This is a not uncommon happening during the aftermath of such devastating news and is well intended:

> I think we were right in retrospect – to take him away and then introduce him to the whole thing once the dust had settled and once all our anxieties and emotions, adult emotions, had subsided . . . then we were able to cope better with introducing [the sibling] to the whole thing saying look [your brother] has cancer we hope he's going to get better.
>
> (Father)

But the effect on the child can be different to the parents' expectations. The sibling in this case appeared to feel isolated and resentful at being sent away, missing school and having to 'get used to' his brother after not being together as a family, however chaotic, at a critical time of their lives.

Other parents appeared to compensate for the lack of verbal communication by spoiling their child, which for this mother seemed to reinforce the pretence that the experience was not real but a bad dream:

> We was buying her everything . . . and what she didn't ask for we got her . . . it was just a complete nightmare . . . we wanted not to do anything, go

anywhere, just to do what she wanted to do. Like wrap her up in cotton wool and think like we're gonna stop here and they're all having us on and kidding us and I'm gonna wake up and things is gonna be alright.

Relationships appeared to be particularly disturbed where the natural parents had divorced whether or not there had been remarriage. The difficulty was not only a matter of being a single parent – of bearing the burden alone, though this was a factor for one mother. The locus of the problem appeared to be that the diagnosis initially tends to be told in the presence of one natural parent (usually the mother) with her current partner if she has one. Consequently the father feels left out, may doubt the facts as relayed by the mother or pick up false facts misperceived by the mother or because of gaps in information. A father said:

I was getting a lot of stuff second hand information you know, which was quite, quite difficult.

Information given to one parent and not another, a situation which at times is unavoidable, can it seems be used as a powerful tool to create conflict in a family already under great pressure. This father admitted to prolonged feelings of gloominess about the prognosis. His mother, the patient's grandmother, put it down to the fact that he had not had the opportunity to speak to the doctors at the time of the diagnosis:

I think we should have been asked to go and see someone at hospital and let someone talk to us like they talked to [the patient's] mum. Getting from her didn't seem the same you know, she had it all from the hospital and they'd reassured her you see that it wasn't as bad as we'd thought it was going to be, it was treatable, and things like that.

Where there was evidence of more open communication, family relationships were reported to become close at this time.

In some ways it brought us closer together because we had a common goal . . . the only way we could get through it was together.

Partners who are able to share their pain, however desolate they feel, can give mutual comfort. But in none of the families was there evidence that all relationships were in balance.

What helped adjustment to the diagnosis?

It is clear from the comments above that both the individual history of the illness and the circumstances in which the parents were told the diagnosis influenced how they adjusted. If the experiences up to this point had been adverse, particularly if they had occurred outside the specialist hospital, the task for the specialist carers to regain their confidence was not easy. It does seem, however, that on arrival at the specialist centre, parents were reassured by the general feeling that they had reached a milestone where they would be given reliable information and some hope for the future.

Major factors which helped adjustment were the provision of information and the way the information was given. Parents felt better when given explanation about the type of cancer, it's causes – reassurance that it wasn't their fault, general understanding and expectations about the disease and its implications in terms of treatment and prognosis, particularly in relation to chances of cure.

Understandably parents felt better if they learnt that the disease was treatable and the patient had a good chance of recovery:

> The doctor told us what she'd got . . . and it was the best cancer to have.
> So I thought that's brilliant that, I mean that really lifted me.

But if the prognosis was not so good, parents appreciated 'the facts as they were', given in a direct, professional and sensitive manner, so they could build up a relationship of trust and confidence. A father who had been disillusioned by the doctors who dealt with their child's care prior to the final diagnosis said the consultant at the specialist hospital had been supportive because:

> She knew her job inside out . . . she was really up front with us and said er, really just sat there and we asked loads of questions which we wanted to ask, and she just sat there, she didn't start looking at her watch, or the usual things you know – I've got this timetable that I have to follow – she just sat there and answered every single question.

Being given time and space and being treated as an individual, 'not a number because everyone has their own fears', were typical remarks about how parents wanted to be treated. Many parents, however, were too much in a state of shock to take anything in at first and, from the evidence above, unwilling or unable to talk or hear what information might be offered. Several mentioned the usefulness of the booklets they were given in this context for both parents (sometimes handed on to grandparents) and a special one for children:

> A booklet to read, to have everything wrote down in front of you, to explain things to us and they gave us an itinery (sic) of what were going to happen to [the patient] all through and it were brilliant, you know everything mapped out perfectly, and you knew exactly what was going off all the time.
>
> (Father)

The expression of relief – of having come through chaos to find the way ahead clearly marked is palpable in this father's comment. It is typical of many. Yet while it is clearly vital to provide this kind of support it is surely equally important to be realistic. The terrain ahead, in many respects, cannot be charted. And it is this inevitable uncertainty of the future that both parents and professional carers found difficulty in dealing with.

The first encounter with the children's cancer ward had a powerful effect on many parents. For some it was supportive and encouraging:

Seeing other families going through the same thing . . .

Seeing a lot worse than your own child . . . talking to them helped . . . they were brilliant.

When you're all in the same boat it's easier.

Conversely there were others who found it distressing:

It was a shock seeing children and babies with cancer . . . I'd not realized children could have cancer.

Walking onto the ward – it was so noisy, overpowering and I thought I hope it's not going to be like this every time.

Most got used to this highly charged atmosphere, but all were affected by the deaths of other children which fuelled their fears for their own child's uncertain future.

Some parents were helped by talking to friends or close relatives, especially if they could share positive experiences of their own – 'The child recovered'; 'Something could be done'. Physical affection was mentioned several times as a help in coping, particularly by mothers:

'Words were not enough. I needed to he held.

One mother who was the breadwinner of the family as her husband was ill said:

Someone to hug me and say 'I'm here for you' would have helped.

Another factor which seemed to help reduce the sense that the world had turned upside down was expressed in a number of different ways as trying to live to as 'normal' a routine as possible. These mothers said:

Well I kept goin' . . . for t' rest of t' family . . . if I hadn't 'a done I'da just fell to pieces.

Keeping busy . . . just every day things you carry on you've got to . . . just getting over every little bit at a time.

For most parents the best help was the sense that the doctors had taken over and were **doing** something and then seeing their child responding to treatment despite the traumas of the treatment itself.

The main dilemma for professional carers engaged in helping families adjust is the parents' need for information and talking things through at a time when they are in a state of shock and unable or unwilling to listen or talk. Parents' ambivalence is understandable for it seems that though they want information and to talk, they would prefer to hear only good news. By avoiding communication they can continue believing this is a bad dream. The implications for practice are possibly to have a professional carer trained in counselling skills available from the moment of diagnosis who can continually assess and monitor the individual needs of each family member.

EFFECT ON NORMAL LIFE

The term 'normal' has, of course, a different meaning for different people. Here its meaning derives from the perspective of the person interviewed. Each member of the family was asked about how their lives changed, how their feelings changed and how they coped with the changes over time.

Table 6.1 Effect on normal life

		N =	Positive	Negative
Fathers	pro	9	3	9
	retro	8	4	32
total		17	7	41
Mothers	pro	10	6	20
	retro	9	6	60
total		19	12	80

Fathers

Most fathers talked of disruption of their normal life in terms of their work. The majority had sympathetic employers, but despite this they spoke of guilt at not being able to be as much with their child or siblings as they wished. One had recently become self-employed and felt bitter and guilty that he couldn't take time off. If he had, he said:

> We would finish up in a worse position 'cos we would have a lot more stress in terms of wondering how we gonna have enough to pay for the house etc.

Another said there had been friction with his employers – time off had to be taken as holiday and no pay. Finally he lost his job.

Several fathers found work a welcome distraction from the constant anxiety. But at the same time they said it was often hard to concentrate:

> It was a big help to me to be able to carry on with me job like well not forget it but you know what I mean, be doin' something else other than thinking about it 90 per cent of the time . . . I mean you never forget about it, I mean every time you pull up at a set of traffic lights you're thinking about will he be alright.

Mothers

The high number of negative aspects reported by mothers (double those of fathers) suggests that they bear the onus of care of patient and family. The fathers are to some extent shielded by the responsibility of resuming work at the earliest opportunity. This does not mean fathers felt less emotional pain, but that their lives tended to be disrupted less.

Mothers were most upset about leaving the care of well siblings in the hands of others – grandparents, other relatives, friends or neighbours – so that they could concentrate on the patient. They were especially distressed if the siblings had to be split up. They felt guilty that the siblings were missing out on attention, and paradoxically annoyed if the grandparent over-indulged them so impeding the return to normal. Common feelings were of torn loyalties; the wish to 'cut meself in half' and the fear of the healthy siblings 'growing away from me' or something happening to them – an accident or illness. One mother felt particularly guilty when she discovered her younger healthy child was deaf and had developed communication difficulties. She felt that had she been giving him due attention the disability would have been identified and attended to earlier and the ensuing difficulty in communication avoided.

They were also upset if they had to leave older siblings to fend for themselves. A mother who's husband had walked out three weeks after the diagnosis (there was already conflict in the marriage) said of her daughter:

> I had to depend on her to look after the house . . . I didn't realize when I think back now that I'd put so much on our Sally. I mean she had to get herself up to go to work [she was aged 16].

On reflection she added that she thought it had brought them closer.

Spoiling of both siblings and patients caused several mothers concern. One mother was quick to see the effects on her son:

> Folks used to be buying 'im things, and giving 'im things an' 'e thought then 'e were gonna die, and that's why folks were doin' it.

Another was straightforward in her response to her child who, taking advantage of the situation, wanted everything doing for him. She said to him:

Do summat for yourself . . . if you don't you're just gonna lie there and
die! . . . I 'ad to be honest wi' 'im. That was the first time 'e knew 'e
could die . . . within a couple of hours 'e was out o' bed walkin' up an'
down! That's all 'e needed. 'E needed honesty.

Four mothers mentioned they had to give up work to look after their ill child.
Whilst they wanted to do this, the loss of income incurred at a time when there
were many additional costs was a major concern. One mother had to subsequently sell their house and move to a smaller one to reduce their cost of living.
Several mentioned the social isolation they experienced. Even relatives would
stay away:

> I sometimes felt as though they couldn't cope with it . . . they didn't want
> to come and see us for weeks . . . they couldn't talk about it.

> I think they were frightened of the hair loss.

> I think they thought it was catching.

Mothers were concerned and distressed by the ignorance they encountered.
They expected a degree of bullying from schoolchildren; they felt deeply for
their child having to cope with it, but were shocked by adults' reactions. One
recalled how people in the street stared at her child's baldness, another how a
friend had crossed the road to avoid talking to her. But another reason for this
isolation was because some mothers were reluctant to go out:

> I was always in, wouldn't let [the patient] leave my side.

This was an understandable feeling of protectiveness, and seemed linked to a
sense of helplessness. This mother was typical:

> You feel useless. If there was any way you could help, but you can't, you
> can't do anything, you just feel useless – absolutely useless. I felt 'Oh
> God I wish it was me'.

Implicit is the sense that at least if I watch over my child constantly I'm doing
something – fulfilling my role as a mother.

Throughout the period after diagnosis and through treatment to the early days
back at home, a period which could last over two years, many mothers felt tired
and run down. In this state of near exhaustion, as one mother put it, 'the imagi-
nation runs riot' and fears and anxieties can become magnified.

Understandably both parents felt their normal lives were affected in a negative way. What is surprising is that there were some positive factors. These were
expressed mainly in terms of family and friends 'rallying around', 'pulling
together', 'becoming closer'.

ADJUSTMENT BACK TO NORMAL

Table 6.2 Adjustment back to normal life

		N =	Positive	Negative
Fathers	pro	9	4	1
	retro	8	1	15
total		17	5	16
Mothers	pro	10	6	20
	retro	9	6	60
total		19	12	80

Fathers

Fathers seemed to take a more general view of life getting back to normal in comparison to the more detailed accounts of mothers. Perhaps simply because they had less to do with the details of returning to normal apart from their own arrangements for work. When asked after his child's treatment had finished, 'How has your life been affected now?' a father replied:

We're normal, we're as normal as can be (laughs) no we're alright, we're sound.

Another said:

It takes a year out of your life, er it's been a strange experience . . . life stops and starts again. I think that's basically how you can say it is, really difficult to explain.

When asked, 'So where do you see yourself now then?' this father replied, with a laugh, 'Oh the world's starting again'.

Fathers seemed particularly moved by the way in which their child had shown such spirit and determination throughout the course of the illness:

How she's accepted it . . . it's been an inspiration . . . it's out of this world, she said 'I'm ready for owt'.

It's as if he said 'I've beat that, now I'm gonna enjoy myself'.

Mothers

Mothers were understandably frightened of leaving the caring and supportive environment of the hospital with the responsibility of day to day care on their shoulders, although for one it had some compensation:

Obviously it's a bit unnerving at first but I was glad to get home and get some sleep.

One mother described a particularly 'horrendous' time when her daughter kept bleeding from the mouth. Others had difficulty feeding their child and were distressed at the speed he or she lost weight. The visual aspects seemed to have contributed most to the mothers' anxiety and they were unable to escape them for long. One mother and daughter became increasingly 'ratty' with each other from being together so much. They talked about it and resolved the situation by the mother going back to work for one day a week when her daughter went back to school.

The main concerns of mothers were associated with the fear of recurrence:

I'm a little bit cautious with him . . . any aches or pains.

I still worry . . . especially if he's playing football ever and he gets banged 'ard, 'cos they say they don't know what starts it off, don't they? Things like that.

Panic sets in when she has a headache.

These fears often lead to overprotectiveness yet with a realization that their child had to learn and wanted to be independent. The struggle to reach a balance was brought to the surface by one parent's exasperated response to his son's wish to buy a motor bike:

We didn't come through all this just for you to get killed on a bike.

A mother in the retrospective group put the change in her feelings in a very clear perspective. She speaks for many:

I feel jumpy with it now. It's like living with a time bomb. You didn't have that while he were having treatment. It's a terrible thing to say, but it was our best time. I felt they were doing something. All the time they were striving to make him better, and now I feel that we're just playing the waiting game to see if it's going to come back.

Looking at the totals of positive and negative comments so far it appears that whilst normal life is disrupted in a negative way adjustment becomes less negative (rather than more positive) which is perhaps to be expected. There is an interesting difference between the prospective and retrospective group however. The fathers, and to a lesser extent the mothers, in the prosepctive group appear to be more optimistic about this stage. The retrospective group looked back on this time with more negative recollections. Whilst this could be because professional carers have improved their skills and resources are more widely available, making the transition to normal life smoother, it was clear to the interviewers that the explanation was more likely to be that respondents in the prospective group were buoyed up by the child's recent response to treatment. For the retrospective group, reflecting from at least two years distance, the concern colouring most recollections was the threat of recurrence.

CHANGES IN LIFE DURING REMISSION

Table 6.3 Changes during remission

		N =	Positive	Negative
Fathers	pro	9	9	9
	retro	8	11	27
total		17	20	36
Mothers	pro	10	7	10
	retro	9	8	32
total		19	15	42

Fathers

Fathers looked at changes in two ways – how the illness had changed their child and how it had changed, in broad terms, their philosophy of life. Some were concerned about the possible permanent side effects of treatment such as sterility and intellectual impairment. One father wondered when it would be appropriate to break the news of possible infertility to his son. Another had had ambitions for his daughter as she had been a clever girl, and now school reported she sometimes had mental blocks following radiotherapy for a brain tumour.

Other aspects of change were noticed in the child's personality. For one father this was negative – 'She's become passive, she never asks questions'. But another was pleased to see a change in his son's attitude to life: 'He seems to enjoy hisself more'. Several said they felt their child had grown up a lot, 'become tougher', 'more assertive', 'confident'. But these changes were two-edged:

I think that all kids that have no matter what kind of cancer . . . for some reason it takes something away from their childhood; they are never . . . they don't seem to be a child anymore.

Both fathers and mothers talked similarly of a changed way of living life, living from day to day, week to week, not taking things for granted, believing anything could happen – which, paradoxically, was for some a positive factor because:

> You're prepared for anything . . . if you've gone through that you can cope with anything.

> It's prepared me for when my time comes, whatever circumstances, because I'm sure I'd be a lot more positive with me own illness.

They describe a new relish for life lived in the present but with major drawbacks:

> I think to meself, don't think about doing things in 10 years, think about doing them now . . . it's made things worse because I tend to spoil [my kids] now a lot worse than I used to . . . you know you would never forgive yourself for not letting them have what they wanted, and do what they want . . . touch wood but anything could happen . . . it could be one or two of them next month, next year.

What it is like living with the fear of recurrence – 'this big question hanging over you' – was summed up by this father:

> I feel I've got to be prepared for any relapse . . . petrol in the car etc. I feel as though it's probably a tightrope I'm on.

Mothers

The experience of childhood cancer seems to be particularly hard on mothers – perhaps predictably since they seem to be the main carers. The rates of positive and negative comments are higher than for fathers and though the negative do reduce over time they remain predominant.

The anxieties about long term effects on their children were similar to those of the fathers including concerns about whether a son's disability might prevent him from following the career of his choice, and whether the visible paralysis of a daughter's face would affect her as she grew up. One mother felt such a failure at producing children – her first died at birth, the second had cancer and the third was deaf – she said:

> I'm petrified of having a baby . . . I blame myself because I can't have a baby in the normal way . . . I just wish I hadn't had children really.

The over-riding fear for all mothers is that of recurrence which manifested itself through constant attention to their child's health – aches and pains; activities – overprotectiveness, 'mollycoddling' and 'spoiling him rotten'. One mother said:

> I don't think I'll ever treat him as normal . . . until he's an old man and dies of old age.

Others described how this fear affected their whole outlook on life:

Because it's not there now it doesn't mean to say that in a week or a fortnight it's not going to move.

I think it's still really the reality that he could still die I don't want to come to terms with.

If I could **see** it had gone I'd be a lot happier.

It's frightening it makes you think you don't know what's going to happen.

You never know what's round the corner.

I allus think my two little ones could grow up and have same happen to them . . . it could come out at any time . . . it always worries me. I'm frightened to think about it.

The uncertainty goes on for weeks, months, years.

It's on our minds 24 hours a day.

These are only a few of many comments showing that the fear is always present to some degree, that it spills over to fear for the health of other siblings. It also does not appear to diminish; indeed for some it worsens as the years pass, as the higher score of negatives in the retrospective group seems to indicate.

Again, however, mothers show how they can transcend the pain of living with the uncertain and sometimes indifferent world they describe. They make of their tragedy a triumph that is more than mere survival:

If we've been through it once, we'll cope again.

Now I worry about other people more than myself really because I know I can cope . . . I've gone through two broken marriages, and then for this to happen, well, it was like a kick in the teeth if you like but it strengthened me, I am a stronger person for it, and I'm stronger for a lot ot people.

The overall pattern of negative and positive aspects indicates that the time immediately after diagnosis was the worst for parents. During treatment anxieties decreased, especially if the patient responded well. The return to 'normal' however, particularly in the retrospective group was marked by a rise again in negative aspects dominated by the overshadowing fear of uncertainty as to what the future holds – a fear largely hidden from specialists (as they now only see the family at check ups) and from the GP (as they have mostly been excluded from care from the time of diagnosis). Parents' fears are also unspoken around their local community as childhood cancer is relatively rare and few would understand. Most people see the child having come through and expect the rest to be 'plain sailing'. Whilst this predominant concern of the precariousness of the future cannot be made to disappear with the wave of a magic wand, intervention should be available for parents at the most vulnerable times to help them emerge from this experience with a better chance of gaining a more positive view of their future.

The Extended Family 7

Your concern is sort of split, you know sort of grandad and parent sort of thing . . . like a dual feeling . . . to a degree you're sort of helpless, you know what can you, what will they let you do. You've got to take that into consideration . . . you can't push yourself in and take over. You've got to sort of stand back and be supportive . . . you're there when you're needed, not interfere, but to help you know . . . it's a difficult bit of balance to get you know.

Grandparents, aunts, uncles, even close friends and neighbours who are often regarded by children as 'auntie' or 'uncle' are inevitably deeply affected when a child they know and love has cancer. Few research studies have explored the feelings of this group, yet it is clear from this grandfather that the effects on those closely involved are complex and finding the best 'balance' in relation to the rest of the family is not easy.

In this study the child with cancer, the parents and siblings were asked who, outside the immediate family, was closely involved and permission to approach them was negotiated. The total number of extended family interviewed was 17 (see Table 7.1).

Table 7.1 The extended family

	Prospective	Retrospective
Grandfathers	4	2
Grandmothers	7	2
Aunts	2	0
Total	13	4

The majority of extended family interviewed were grandparents and this chapter focuses on this special relationship in the family. However, although the term 'grandparent' is used throughout, it should be read as representative of the perspective of this group including anyone who is seen by the family as an integral part of their lives.

Many of the effects experienced by grandparents were similar to those of the parents. They felt the same devastation, shock and numbness when they heard the diagnosis, with the attendant disbelief that cancer could strike children. They were distressed to see their grandchild go through treatment which made them so ill and yet carried no guarantee of cure. Similarly there were persistent fears of recurrence of the disease. Because of these similarities in the way the experience changed their lives and also because the numbers are relatively small, this chapter will not dwell on comparing the estimates of positive and negative comments as in the previous chapter. Enough to say that the results for grandfathers mirror those of fathers and those of grandmothers mirror the mothers. The focus here will be on the differences: the way in which the special relationship of grandparent is affected from the perspectives of all the family members, and the positive and negative factors that flow from the fact that they are predominantly elderly.

THE DIAGNOSIS

The fact that a child can have cancer is a particularly poignant burden for a grandparent to bear:

> Why a bairn . . . you just think of cancer in old people, you don't realize that young people can get it.

All the factors discussed in Chapter 2 on the meaning of cancer were raised frequently by grandparents: that it couldn't affect the young; that their grandchild had been so healthy – running around so full of life only yesterday; that it couldn't be happening to us; that it should be me – if only I could bear it for him or her. The sense of loss of childhood and the unfairness of the order of things was very strong:

> He was only a little boy and you thought well something serious at his age . . . you don't know how to cope quite, all you can do is hope and pray . . . you don't know who is going to be next . . . all the way through life. You couldn't believe it that little babies and little kids like could suffer so . . . they'd done nothing wrong in their lives to deserve it.

One reason why the feelings of disbelief and confusion were particularly marked was possibly because grandparents mostly heard the diagnosis second hand, usually from the parents who would have been themselves in a state of shock and may not have taken in details of prognosis and treatment. Such information, when it does sink in, alleviates the worst fears and provides some understanding, structure and above all hope for the future. It cannot be quite the same for grandparents to have it relayed to them from their children as it is for the parents to hear it from the lips of the consultant, a group respected by all parents. One father even referred to the consultant as a 'god', such was his faith in her ability to treat his son.

CHANGES IN RELATIONSHIP

The grandparents in several families, and one aunt, looked after siblings and at times the patient when out of hospital, to give the parents respite. Many contributed in practical ways such as taking on the ironing or cooking meals for older siblings on their return from school. For some this was hard due to disablement, poor health or simply the amount of 'toing and froing'. Or they found the behaviour of the child, whether sibling or patient, difficult to handle:

> She were gettin' a bugger through it . . . I just more or less gi'd 'er all 'er own road. I suffered for it later . . . she got to point where she wouldn't take no for an answer . . . I don't think I'd make that mistake again wi' 'er.

Others clearly surmounted all the physical drawbacks of their advanced age with small triumphs of diplomacy and wisdom. One set of grandparents took their grandchild with them on a caravan holiday and had to deal with difficulties of eating problems due to the after effects of chemotherapy and teasing from children on the caravan site who made fun of the boy's bald head and emaciated features. The grandparents solved the first problem with a constant supply of the child's favourite Yorkshire puddings and onion gravy, and the second by talking to the parents of the teasing children explaining the reason for his appearance. When understanding had been reached, the families became good friends and the children played happily together for the rest of the holiday.

Grandparents found it difficult not to spoil their grandchildren – perhaps a common tendency which is exacerbated by the circumstances. Some were aware of it even to the extent that they knew it was upsetting the parents. One grandmother admitted:

> I drove her parents crazy, me grandchild had to have everything.

This grandmother was exceptional in her obsessive negative feelings – nothing and no one could convince her that her grandchild was responding to treatment. She couldn't sleep, lost weight, rejected the rest of her numerous grandchildren, had no time for her husband who was frail and had recently had a small stroke. Her grandchild's illness, she said, 'took over me life . . . I were oblivious to everything'. Most were less extreme in their response to the situation and would agree with this grandparent's explanation for their partial behaviour:

> I've relived me life through me grandchildren . . . different than with your own children . . . I couldn't do for me own kids what I could for me grandkids.

Another grandmother said:

> Grandchildren are different . . . you've got more time for them.

Having more time is clearly a positive factor if grandparents are able to use it to help out parents with childcare, but it has a negative side besides spoiling. The relationship, particularly between maternal grandmother and mother (mother/daughter), was sometimes strained. With more time on their hands they were preoccupied with anxieties about the ill grandchild. For example one daughter said her mother 'pestered' her with phone calls at least once a day to find out how the child was, another pressed her to check with the doctor every time her child had a fall, or cautioned her to keep the child indoors in bad weather – they seemed to want continual information on their grandchild's progress and reassurance that he or she was alright but never quite dared to believe the news when it was good.

One grandmother went as far as blaming the mother (her daughter-in-law) for neglecting her child and being the cause of delayed diagnosis and subsequent slow recovery. The parents stopped visiting them, but the grandparents continued to see their ill grandchild, plying her with presents and extra pocket money, meanwhile ignoring the well grandchild. The effects on family relationships were divisive and long lasting, particularly affecting the well grandchild (see Chapter 5 on siblings), despite both parents' efforts to keep communications open and honest between the immediate family.

Not all interference from grandparents was seen in such a negative light. One mother recalled how she and her husband were intensely angry and blaming each other when they first heard their son had cancer. It took some firm but gentle prompting from her mother-in-law to help them see that for the sake of both their children 'the only way through was together . . . we went back to loving each other just the same as we did . . . in some ways it brought us closer together'. The well sibling in this family received much care from her grandparents and said it made them all much closer. She was not alone in enjoying living for a while with close relatives. A sibling who had a single mother was sent to her auntie, just down the road, to stay whilst her brother was in hospital. She said:

> It were great – playing with me cousins . . . I thought it were brill – it were a luxury more than anything.

The success of this arrangement may be partly due to the fact that the auntie lived close by and the sibling could remain at the same school and continue close contact with her family and friends. In another family a sibling was sent some distance away to an aunt and appeared to miss knowing first hand what was going on with his brother and events at school which he was unable to attend during this time.

SPECIFIC CONCERNS

It is clearly expressed in the opening quotation that a grandparent's concern is divided between their child and their grandchildren. Most were aware of the tremendous strain on the parents which they felt helpless to alleviate:

> She got really low, although she never complained or anything like that . . . she never left him . . . it must be draggin' her down.

> It's the effect it has on others that bounces back and hits yer . . . the main thing [was] it really did hit [my daughter] well and truly hard you know.

Perhaps because they often had more contact with the siblings than the parents they seemed particularly aware of how the experience was affecting them. One grandfather was most upset that the younger siblings had to be split up for childcare while the patient was in hospital. Another said 'his little life was shattered' and they tried to offset this by ferrying him home so he could sleep in his own bed at the end of each day he was in their care, despite it being more tiring for them – the grandfather was disabled by back trouble which gave him more or less constant pain.

The health of the grandparents was an additional concern of parents. Two families said that soon after their child had been diagnosed the grandfather had a stroke. In one it was directly related to the shock and distress of the experience, but the other, it was suggested, was one of a series of mild strokes suffered in the last few years. The consequences for the parent were similar, however: 'I felt torn in two – who do you visit?'. The fact that the treatment of childhood cancer extends over several years means that inevitably major concurrent events occur, such as another close family member's illness or death, draining the family's already taxed physical and emotional resources still further.

Perhaps a positive aspect of a grandparent's precarious health is illustrated by one grandmother who had been seeing her GP regularly for high blood pressure. Soon after she heard the diagnosis her blood pressure soared. Her doctor asked what she thought might have caused the sudden rise and on hearing the news allowed her to express her fears and was always willing to listen on subsequent visits to the surgery. The fact that the elderly are more likely to see their family doctor more often than the rest of the family, who are predominantly under the specialist's care, can provide grandparents with a valuable support system. Furthermore it provides the family doctor, if he attends to the rest of the family's care, a perspective on the state of their welfare.

VIEWS OF THE FUTURE

Grandparents seemed to have great insight into the experience of childhood cancer, manifesting a particularly integrated yet holistic view of the family. Perhaps this is because they were one step removed and because of their overview of three generations. Whatever the reason it is a perspective of great value to the family when used to help each member see and communicate their disparate needs and work together to support each other. Their insight is also a gift to researchers, providing a strong argument for taking the extra trouble and expense of including the extended family in a study which aims to focus on complex family issues.

Their insight, however, was costly to themselves. Their fears of recurrence of the cancer were as great as those of the parents:

> It's one of those things that I don't think you ever get over, even though she's better. I can be ironing and I can think oh good grief I hope that don't come up again because it would kill me it really would.

In addition to their concern for their grandchild's health they feared even more what would happen to all the family if they had to go through the experience again.

There is an awareness that life has changed for everyone – in a moment of sudden realization a grandfather said of his grandson, now in remission:

> I just treat 'im as normal . . . well as normal . . . you can't treat 'im as normal'.

And a grandmother observed that the family had talked a lot together when the patient was first diagnosed and during treatment but not subsequently about the illness. Whilst this is perhaps understandable, as many said once the patient became stronger they wanted to put the experience behind them, it may explain why residual problems of any member of the family, but particularly the needs of the siblings, can remain suppressed and concealed.

A more positive change was observed by a grandmother who had been very concerned about the amount of spoiling her granddaughter had had:

> I thought she would grow up wanting this and wanting the other . . . but she's grown up immensely, she's taking everything in her stride.

And a grandfather felt his grandson's outlook on life had changed:

> It's done him good in that way . . . he's a happy go lucky lad now.

An interesting contrast of perspectives of the future from two grandmothers in the same family shows how both positive and negative responses can co-exist. The paternal grandmother was unusually pessimistic and reflected that she'd rather her granddaughter had been killed in a car crash than have cancer, since she was condemned to live with the continual fear of recurrence:

I know that would be a terrible tragedy but now I'm at the stage where I'm driving [my daughter-in-law] crackers with regard to what I'm saying to her . . . it's making me paranoid.

The maternal grandmother had nursed her husband with cancer until his death not long before her grandaughter was diagnosed. She said when considering the changes the experience of her grandaughter's illness had wrought on their lives:

It's made [the parents] realize [their daughter] is there which they are very glad for with all the help and care they've had and also made them realize that things can happen any time with any one of them. So you've just got to sort of take step by step. You see my motto is now take every day as it comes and thank God for it.

The grandfather who posed the dilemma of the grandparents' role with such insight and sensitivity at the beginning of this chapter now ends it with a philosophy evoked as he looked back, and to an extent, relived the pain and suffering he had experienced during his grandson's illness:

Time's a great healer, I've always believed that, and eventually things do become I wouldn't say distant but softer. You can look back and there's that many things that have taken place in between that they soften with the distance. You can sort of look back and it doesn't hit you so hard. The more you look back and go through the events, you'll never forget, it's impossible to forget but it does become easier. When there's a bereavement or anything it takes your heart, you want to bring them back, but over the years it eases off, it's a similar thing in a way.

8	# Professional Carers: The Emotional Costs

Professional carers who work with families where a child has cancer have to face the demands of working in a highly emotive environment. This can at times be difficult, yet it is not without its rewards. Several studies have attempted to explore the specific issues that are raised when health professionals work with families where a child has a life-threatening illness (Lansdown and Goldman, 1988; Wooley *et al.*, 1989). The focus of this work has concentrated on how professionals cope with death and dying. Few studies address the emotional costs of helping families live with uncertainty and the implications that this cost has for care.

In this study health professionals working in both the hospital and community were interviewed. The interviews provided the opportunity to explore their experiences and perceptions in relation to working with children who have cancer, and their families. Analysis of the interviews revealed many themes which highlighted the complexities of the issues affecting health professionals working with these families. The main themes identified were:

- negative and positive aspects of the work;
- attitudes to breaking bad news;
- helping families adjust to uncertainty;
- emotional costs of the work;
- coping strategies of health professionals.

NEGATIVE AND POSITIVE ASPECTS OF THE WORK

Ability to handle a challenging situation

Situations were described as difficult when health professionals felt that they could not cope with a specific situation. The same situation could be described as a positive aspect of the work if the member of staff felt that he or she had dealt with it well. For example, families that were seen to be both difficult and challenging were those where conflict existed, where there had been divorce or separation perhaps. In these situations the emotive nature of childhood cancer is intensified by conflict within the family, with 11 hospital-based staff describing difficulties in this area. One nurse spoke of how she felt working with a recon-stituted family who were finding it hard to talk openly about the diagnosis:

> . . . Dad still didn't want to tell him . . . [the patient] . . . Mum did want to tell him. And, er, things were getting very uptight. You could feel the undercurrents as soon as you walked on the ward . . . it all came out . . . when they had a talk with the social workers, doctors, Mum and Dad, Dad's new partner and the nursing staff. . .'

The nurse found working with this family very difficult. It left her feeling ' . . . really . . . very out of my depth . . .'.

Similar difficulties were described in effectively giving information to family members, so that all were involved and conflict avoided. One nurse explained this by saying:

> . . . You do tread on eggshells at times . . . obviously if you have told one of the parents something then you need to make sure that you tell the other one . . . [if not they may turn round and say] . . . you are telling my ex-partner far more than you are telling me . . . I have an absolute right to know what's going on. Which of course they have. You know so it is stressful at times in that situation.

Relationships

Health professionals saw relationships with colleagues as a particularly reward-ing part of the work. This included comments about the working atmosphere which allowed expression of feelings such as sadness, humour, anger and conflict. Teamwork was also seen as a positive and supportive part of the job which enabled staff to become more involved with families, thus improving the quality of care given.

The negative aspects of relationships included that of role definition. For example, the social workers felt that their role was not always understood by other members of the team, especially medical staff, with the result of role over-lap. Similarly, general practitioners felt concerned about their role, being unsure of their part in supporting these families. One GP expressed this by saying:

> I suspect I have not had enough contact with them ... [the family] ... I suspect that there are problems on both sides, erm I don't know whether I ought to have been, whether I had anything else to offer from what was being already offered ...

Lack of clarity concerning role left some GPs with feelings of guilt as they questioned whether they had done enough to help the family. Another GP commented that before being interviewed for the study,

> . . . I suddenly thought well that kid had cancer and I did nothing you know, all I did I went round and once or twice and I said are you alright . . . and there's a bit of me that felt sort of should I have done more . . .

Involvement

When asked what they found the most rewarding aspect of their work, the majority of the hospital-based staff mentioned the joy of working with children. One nurse said:

> . . . The kids are what really make it . . . some of them will come up and give you a cuddle or . . . draw you a picture . . . and just little things. It's often really little things like that just giving you a picture . . .

Another said, when asked what the rewards were for her,

> ... The children really. They're amazing. I mean there's always going to be those that just grab hold of your heart ...

The intensity of involvement between professionals and families sometimes required the necessity to stand back from the situation. But the social workers, in particular, said that this was not always possible, and described the resultant stress which was exacerbated by a perceived lack of support from colleagues.

A central issue in what were perceived as negative and positive areas of the work was the general theme of communication, and the emotive nature of working with families where a child has cancer.

Staff considered dealing with issues such as collusion difficult. If parents did not want their child to know of a poor prognosis staff found this very stressful as they felt unable to be open and honest with the child. Senior members of staff tried to deal with collusion by helping the parents to see the value of open communication. When applied successfully they found this approach very satisfying.

The impact of the emotive nature of this work was most poignantly expressed by the transient staff. One student nurse admitted feeling overwhelmed when confronted with strong feelings such as anger. She described feeling 'like a chocolate fireguard . . .' when first on the ward in the presence of intense emotions. The more experienced staff were aware of the emotional intensity of the work, however they had developed coping strategies which enabled them to distance themselves from it. Table 8.1 summarizes positive and negative aspects of the work.

Table 8.1 Positive and negative aspects of the work

Positive	Negative
Handling a situation well	Handling a situation badly
United families	Conflict in families
Information well received	Information giving problems
Work atmosphere	Poor role definition
Support from colleagues	Perceived lack of support
Teamwork	Role overlap
Involvement with families	Family emotions – risk of overload

BREAKING BAD NEWS

Breaking bad news was reported as an emotionally charged situation, particularly at initial diagnosis where parents immediately thought that their child would die. It was recognized that the impact of the bad news upon the family was influenced by a number of factors. GPs are often involved in the early stages of diagnosis, and nine out of ten said that this put them in a very difficult position. Childhood cancer is rare and unexpected, the symptoms are often vague, and GPs do not want to over-react. When cancer is diagnosed, it may appear that they failed to act quickly enough, so jeopardizing their relationship with the family. Different opinions were expressed about the effect of being referred to the ward before a final diagnosis was made. Two hospital-based staff felt that by coming on to the ward families were warned about the seriousness of the illness and therefore able to prepare themselves for the diagnosis. Others felt that seeing so many sick children is a shock for families and can be distressing. Once nurse said,

> Seeing the other children . . . they've all got cancer of some description, and the bald heads . . . the minute they walk through the door, has an immediate impact . . .

Health professionals recognized that the time leading up to diagnosis may be very stressful for families and could influence the way that they respond to bad news,

Breaking bad news is not without its emotional cost to the carer. Two of the nurses spoke of how stressful it can be to support families with a newly diagnosed child. A senior doctor said in relation to relapse, i.e. unexpected bad news,

> Thankfully it doesn't happen very often but that is always much more devastating, for me I think, to have to break the news to the family who thought things were going on alright and you realized, on the basis of a blood count or on the basis of an x-ray, that things are not alright.

ADJUSTMENT TO UNCERTAINTY

Working with families where a child has cancer requires help for them to come to terms with the diagnosis. The challenge then changes from breaking bad news to helping families live with an uncertain future. All the health professionals in hospital and community were aware that an uncertain future presented difficulties for the families, yet little emphasis was made in terms of helping families cope with the long term impact of this disease.

Health professionals tended to focus on the medical perspective of the child's disease. They accepted the emotiveness of the risk of relapse but felt that eventually this risk decreases and is seen to be comparable to that of other risks in life, such as having a car accident. Most professionals used a medical model of care to help these families, making it difficult for the long term psychosocial needs of families to be addressed.

Helping families to cope with uncertainty was given a low priority by the majority of health professionals. Seventeen (of 28) said that most of their emotional energy was given to children who were ill or dying and their families. This low priority appeared to be due to feelings of helplessness and discomfort, and could be seen as a coping strategy for health professionals.

Although helping families live with uncertainty was given a low priority, the health professionals had developed some strategies for support, one hospital doctor suggesting that it was important to acknowledge the families' fears and to be honest with them. He felt that rationalizing or offering reassurance was of little value. The social workers too saw the need for families to be able to express their feelings about uncertainty. They said it was important to listen to families and allow them to express their deepest concerns. One nurse said that she tried to help families cope with uncertainty by focusing on positive factors. She acknowledged that, while this could help families, it definitely helped her. She felt that having constantly to accept the threat of death, even with well children, would be too much for her to handle. There was considerable ambiguity about the role that the primary health care team should play in the care of these families while they adjusted to a diagnosis of cancer and an uncertain future.

The GPs, for example, felt that their role was limited in that the families had been 'taken over' by the hospital. However they felt that it was right, to some extent, for the hospital to be directive in that they had the knowledge and skill lacking in the surgeries. Nine GPs felt that they wanted to be more involved with care of the families, and eight of the hospital-based staff were aware that their control of the child's medical care for prolonged periods of time had implications for their long term follow up in the community. The hospital staff acknowledged the need to place greater emphasis on involving the primary health care team.

Three of the hospital-based staff, while recognizing that there is a need for more contact with the GPs, said that the most important part of their role was that of supporting families when a child is dying. Six GPs also stressed this aspect of their role. This reflects the tendency to place more emphasis on caring for families where the child is going to die rather than survive. The ambiguity about the role of the primary health care team centred around two issues:

● their role in care in the community; and
● relationships between community and hospital.

Both the hospital-based staff and the GPs focused on the medical aspects of care in the community, stressing 'immunization', 'specialist information' and the technical interest in long term follow up. Suggestions were made on how to improve relationships between hospital and community, each suggesting the other make the first move, or that more liaison staff were needed (see Chapter 9).

The lack of clarity surrounding the role of the GPs and communication with the hospital seemed to mask the underlying issue of how the health professionals coped with the emotional costs of this type of work. In terms of communication with the hospital one GP said that although the information was good it tended to be 'clinical' and 'impersonal'. He went on to say that it would be better to have a voice on the telephone. Another GP said that to survive it was necessary 'to be an actor'. A third felt that 'it was much better to be a spectator on the sidelines' for his own emotional protection. Comments such as these suggest that ambiguity about roles and relationships between health professionals can be used as alibis. Use of alibis can mean that the health professionals fail to confront the issues of how people working in different settings can acknow-ledge and manage the complex emotional reactions that **they** experience in this type of work.

EMOTIONAL COSTS

It has been seen that the demands made upon professionals who are working with families where a child has cancer, give some indication of the emotional cost to carers. Health professionals identified several aspects of their work which carried an emotional cost (summarized in Table 8.2).

Table 8.2 Areas of work with high emotional cost

Children facing death	– unexpectedness
	– suffering
	– unfairness
	– visual manifestations
Family distress	– helplessness
	– overt emotion
	– identification
	– perceived guilt
Own distress	– personal involvement
	– exhaustion
	– effects on functioning at work and home
	– emotional discharge
	– responsibility for effects of treatment

Children Facing Death

The health professionals in the study felt that working with children facing death could be emotionally draining. There were several reasons for this. Serious illness and death of children is rare in our society and thus unexpected. Simply seeing children suffer was found to be distressing. This was particularly so if there were visual manifestations of the disease or treatment. Accompanying these feelings there was a sense of injustice. It did not seem fair that children should suffer and miss out on a 'normal' childhood.

Family Distress

Seeing parents or children who were upset was often distressing for staff. At times there was a sense of helplessness at not being able to take the distress away. One nurse spoke of feeling helpless at the time of diagnosis because of

> . . . just knowing what they've got to go through and just how difficult it can be . . .

Another found herself identifying with the family's distress as

> Whatever the situation, if you see a couple of people just sobbing, upset, you can't but feel, you know, oh! a lump in your throat, can you?

The impact of this emotion on professionals led to feelings of guilt. For example, a nurse felt concerned that on occasions she had not been able to say 'the right thing' to family members.

Professionals' own distress

The health professionals spoke of times when they felt overwhelmed by the emotional intensity of their work. This affected their personal as well as professional lives. A social worker explained this by saying:

> Well I think that at the lowest moments . . . you risk becoming not just physically exhausted but emotionally exhausted and then you are not able to function as effectively as you would like either in your professional work or your personal life . . .

Maintaining a balance between the pressures of work and a home life was seen to be important. One nurse explained her awareness of the difficulties that can occur if this balance is upset.

> If things are going on at work you get extra sensitive about things at home, you know, you burst into tears . . . if you think about it it's because you're upset about something from work. And vice versa really. If things

are not so good at home . . . or with the family, then it makes you extra sensitive at work.

The distress felt was intensified by the ethical dilemmas presented by the limitations of medical knowledge and public expectations. A senior doctor spoke of feeling the weight of responsibility due to possible unknown side effects that would only become apparent as children survive longer. The doctor said:

> . . . The chickens may come home to roost in the future when we see what damage we have caused with the treatment as they get older . . .

The same doctor found that, with increased experience, it became more difficult to talk to parents. Parents often wanted to try any possible medical intervention even though in some situations further treatment would do more harm than good. The doctor explained this by saying:

> I find that talking to parents doesn't get any easier, it gets harder . . . The longer you're in this game the more you're basing your assessment of the situation on your own experience rather than second hand experience . . . the enthusiasm that you have when you start out for having a go at everything gradually gets tempered with realism and maturity. I find that now I'm more often in the position where I'm trying to persuade parents that we should **not** do something rather than we should do something and I find that an extremely hard thing to do.

COPING STRATEGIES

Despite the emotional intensity of this work the health professional had developed and identified coping strategies (summarized in Table 8.3). Distancing was seen to be a particularly useful coping strategy. The conscious use of mechanisms such as rationalizing enabled the health professionals to adopt some degree of objectivity. One doctor spoke of emphasizing that it is not your child:

> . . . It does affect you personally to some extent but it's not your child, it's not your family . . . I think that one has to be on guard against becoming so involved that you feel it's your loss rather than theirs. But that's partly a self-protective mechanism.

Other strategies were used to help put things in perspective such as visiting the clinics to see well children and focusing on the positive value of caring.

Developing competence was recognized as a means of coping with the more demanding aspects of the work. Transient staff in the hospital said that they found the emotional intensity of the work awesome, partly because they did not know how to deal with the difficulties that arose. Staff who had worked in this area for longer felt that by gaining more experience they developed skills which helped them handle difficulties, this in turn helped them cope.

Table 8.3 Coping strategies to balance high emotional costs

Distancing	– reality perspective
	– no over-involvement
	– seeing well children
	– positive aspects of care
Competence	– gaining experience
	– gaining confidence
Support	– teamwork
	– sharing concerns
	– interaction with colleagues
	– 'balance' in family life
	– friendship networks
	– knowing own strengths

Support from colleagues and family was seen to be a particularly valuable means of coping. Teamwork was considered to be a way of offering support in the working environment. Five GPs mentioned the value of sharing concerns with colleagues. Ten hospital-based staff spoke of feeling able to express emotions and concerns in team meetings. This along with sharing feelings with colleagues on an individual level was found to be very useful. The social workers emphasized the value of peer support from members of the same discipline. This helped them to evaluate their work, set limits and put things in perspective.

Personal support outside of work was seen to be particularly important. The health professionals stressed the need to have a balanced life so that family and friends can be supportive but to avoid 'eroding' the quality of these relationships with work stresses. Self-awareness and being able to set personal limits were also seen to be important.

THE EMOTIONAL COST TO CARERS: IMPACT ON FAMILIES

The coping strategies used by the health professionals enabled them to work effectively in emotionally demanding situations. The impact of these strategies on the families varied, with some adding to the quality of care given whilst others could detract from it.

Strategies which enabled professionals to share feelings and increase their self-awareness, such as teamwork and personal support outside of work, enhanced their ability to care. One nurse commented how teamwork enabled her to improve relationships with families as she felt able to express her feelings in a safe environment. Similarly personal support outside of work was seen by carers to be especially useful in enabling them to maintain a balance and put things in perspective. Again this support enabled professionals to improve their relationships with families.

Developing competence, particularly in the area of communication, was seen to be a very effective strategy in enabling health professionals to cope and also in helping them to improve the quality of care given. However if health professionals have not been able to develop competence due to lack of experience or opportunities to take part in further training, the quality of care they are able to give is inevitably affected.

Three of the hospital-based professionals who had been working in this area for a short time spoke of the difficulties they faced in relation to communication. A particular problem was seen to be communicating with the patient. One felt more comfortable talking to younger children, the other two were more at ease with older children. One of the health professionals commented that the patients were more likely to talk to their parents than the doctors or nurses. However as has been discussed earlier (see Chapters 4 and 5) it is not uncommon for role reversal to occur. In this situation the child and parents may find it difficult to talk openly about what is happening. One teenage patient from the retrospective part of the study spoke of how he developed his understanding of his illness:

Interviewer:	Was there a point later that you understood more about what the disease meant?
Patient:	That was more when I went into the Children's Hospital for radiotherapy and chemotherapy. That were just a ward for cancer and leukaemia sufferers so I could see more what the doctors would say.
Interviewer:	So that was more picked up rather than actually being told?
Patient:	Yes.

Comments such as these from patients suggest that if health professionals feel unable to communicate effectively with children, such inadequacies will not necessarily be compensated for by parents. This scenario implies that use of an effective coping strategy such as undertaking further training in communication skills can directly improve the care that families receive. If health professionals do not have the opportunity to develop experience and skills the ability of families to understand the illness and communicate openly will be reduced. Health professionals commented that distancing helped them to continue to provide care in emotionally charged situations. However, use of this strategy seemed to affect the health professionals' perception and understanding of families' needs. This was most apparent in terms of families' needs in relation to coping with an uncertain future once the child was deemed to be in long term remission.

Hospital-based professionals commented on how seeing children who were in remission in the outpatient clinic helped them to put things in perspective. Parents said that follow up visits to the hospital were very stressful. It made them remember all that they had been through and reinforced the possibility of relapse. One mother said '. . . I dread going to the hospital . . . you know in case anything else cropped up . . .' Another spoke of her feelings about follow up visits:

> I think once them visits are . . . done with, I might feel much better in meself . . . 'Cos it's still . . . well, still a deep reminder when 'e 'as to go back. I know it's just for 'is blood check like and . . . just checking, but . . . I worry.

Whilst health professionals were able to understand the stress on families during periods of illness and treatment they found it more difficult to see the pressure that families experienced coping with long term uncertainty. A senior hospital doctor felt that families were gradually able to understand the risk of remission in quite realistic terms. The GPs made similar comments. One suggested that '. . . as time goes on it gradually becomes easier . . .' The families, however, spoke of the increasing burden of living with uncertainty. One mother from the retrospective group said:

> It's one of those things you never get over, even though she's better, it's always at the back of your mind, always.

Whilst use of distancing as a coping strategy can help health professionals to put things into perspective, however, the negative impact of this strategy is that it can make it more difficult for professionals to understand the families' perspectives and needs.

CONCLUSION

Three major conclusions arise from this part of the study. First there is the paradox that those elements of the work which have a negative effect on some are identical to those that are seen as positive by others. The key appears to be in education, and breaking bad news can be seen to be an example of this. Those professionals who had learned strategies to break bad news found the task far less distressing than those who had not. This links with the findings of Faulkner (1992) who showed that few health professionals have been taught to interact effectively with patients and relatives. It is argued here that further training in interactive skills could improve job satisfaction and as a result the standards of care given.

Secondly, support was seen as an important element in coping. This is another area of health care where too little emphasis is put on setting up adequate support mechanisms. 'Burnout' (Burnard 1991) is an accepted phenomenon, but concern for health professionals' survival remains a low priority. A first step would be more honesty in the team of the cost of caring, and permission to admit to that cost.

Finally, much work is required to improve relationships between the hospital and community staff. It is obvious that each sees the other's point of view but there appears to be little commitment to working towards change. Acknowledging the emotion experienced by health professionals in this setting is an important step in improving relationships between the hospital and community. Caring for children with cancer and their families is at once rewarding, frustrating and emotionally draining. It would appear that it could be more rewarding with adequate education, support and commitment to improved relationships between hospital and community. Improving job satisfaction and relationships between teams can only add to the quality of care that families receive.

REFERENCES

Burnard, P. (1991) Beyond burn-out. *Nursing Standard,* **5** (43), 46–8.

Faulkner, A. (1992) The evaluation of training programmes for communication skills in palliative care. *Journal of Cancer Care*, **1** (2), 75–8.

Lansdown, R. and Goldman, A. (1988) The psychological care of children with malignant disease. *Journal of Child Psychology and Psychiatry*, **29** (5), 555–67.

Wooley, H., Stein, A., Forest, G. and Baum, J. (1989) Cornerstone care for families of children with life threatening illness. Personal communication.

9 | Collaboration between Carers

> There's often an assumption from our side that [the family] are thoroughly involved with the hospital and an assumption from the hospital that they get support elsewhere and that can be a problem . . . there's a bit of me that feels I should have done more.
>
> (General practitioner)

The improved prognosis for children with cancer poses new challenges for professional carers. In the past, when most children died, professional care was largely in the hands of the specialists, GPs would be involved only if the child died at home. Now more children spend shorter periods in hospital, more can be treated as outpatients and more can expect to return to their 'normal' patterns of life – a transition which may last several years.

The new challenge for professional carers is to help families to **live** with cancer from the moment of diagnosis, through the difficult stages of adjustment to treatment and, during the ensuing years, to cope with the resultant uncertainty. How this can be achieved and by whom remains a matter for debate and resolution. The specialists have clinical expertise in what is a relatively rare disease and the opportunity to work with the family to build up trust and confidence through months and perhaps years of treatment. The GP and the primary health care team may have known the family for years and feel a special responsibility for the reintegration of the family unit into the local community. One could argue that both the specialist and the primary health care team have a distinct role in the care of a family where a child has cancer. In reality, it is not uncommon for there to be problems in terms of role and function of those involved with the family.

In this chapter the views of professional carers, both GPs and specialists, are explored to consider the role and function of GPs in providing care for children with cancer and their families, and the relationship of those GPs to the specialist carers. Ten GPs were interviewed who were involved in caring for families included in the research study where the patient was currently or had recently completed treatment. From the specialist perspective, 18 doctors, nurses and social workers, who all worked in the regional paediatric oncology unit of a children's hospital, were interviewed. They varied in seniority and length of experience they had in cancer care.

THE GP's ROLE

All the GPs interviewed agreed that clinical control of the child's disease had to be in the hands of specialists:

> Specialists are the only people who can deal with things . . . [the child] has to be treated at a regional centre.

The difficulty with this was that GPs were then left unsure of their role in relation to what was provided for the child and family at the hospital:

> I was left wondering if I was needed – meant to be involved but wasn't for some reason.

> I don't know whether I could be helpful or not – that's the trouble.

One GP felt regret that a family in his practice had not sought his help. To explain his lack of involvement he tried to look at the situation through the eyes of the family:

> There were a lot of people involved and I suspect they felt there was not much for me actually to do . . . I suspect they didn't look at their own needs.

Specialist views were more variable. As one consultant put it:

> GPs and primary health care teams come in all shapes and sizes and some are much more actively involved and want to be involved than others. Some clearly want to have nothing to do with it.

Five specialists felt it depended on the quality and length of the relationship the GP had with the family, and how the GP had handled the pre-diagnosis stage:

> . . . [the family] often have negative feelings about the GP because nine times out of ten he was their first port of call.

This is an important factor in the relationship between family and their doctor to consider. Early symptoms are often vague, making any delays appear to be the fault of the GP. Seven out of ten interviewed were involved at the diagnosis stage and the parents of only one family changed their doctor because they were dissatisfied and angry about the way he had handled the pre-diagnosis stage of their child's illness. Complaints by both parents and GPs of misdiagnosis and delays were more often laid at the door of the District General Hospital. One family doctor who had worked in paediatric oncology in the past, suspected that his patient, who had presented with a swelling on his shin, had a leukaemic deposit. In his referral to the local hospital he requested that the x-ray should be seen by somebody senior. He later received a message from a locum registrar saying 'No fracture seen'. It was only much later that he had a report saying 'Strongly support leukaemic deposit'. At interview he said:

> I was furious, well by which time [the patient's parents] had got more concerned and they by-passed us completely and had gone to [the specialist] . . .

It is unusual for GPs to have specialist knowledge of diagnosing childhood cancer but it was found that most were concerned about the way in which the period before diagnosis was handled. They were aware of the possible consequences that a delayed diagnosis had on their future relationship with the family, several expressing regret at not having enabled a speedier route to specialist care. A typical reflection on this difficult stage of the family history was this doctor's retrospective scrutiny of her patient's first presentation:

> I feel I possibly was at fault at not getting her seen even faster than I did . . . but then even the consultant ophthalmologist didn't recognize the fact that it was a tumour, but then perhaps we can all criticize ourselves at this level. I mean I did arrange for her to have an appointment as soon as I could but I perhaps should have been more aware of the possibility of it being a cerebral tumour . . . but then I've been in practice 25 years and it's only the third [case of childhood cancer] I've had.

The family had no complaints about this doctor's handling of any stage of their child's illness.

Several specialists believed that the family doctor did not want to be involved but admitted that this was not one sided, for example:

> There ought to be more involvement . . . but sometimes we avoid them and they avoid us.

There was also some variation and ambivalence about what was considered the appropriate degree of involvement. One GP described his role as 'minor', another as 'passive' with no clinical control over treatment. He added that this was appropriate but his ambivalence was evident:

> The problem with childhood cancers are that they are rarely dealt with by the GP, they are jealously guarded by the specialist, I think for very good reason, because only they have sufficient daily ongoing knowledge to be able to deal with the finer aspects of survival . . . we just don't have those skills.

Although, at a logical level, all carers agreed that control of treatment should reside with the specialists, this caused problems for eight out of ten GPs interviewed who felt excluded. 'Sidetracked', 'Bypassed', 'Cut out of the action' were some of the terms typically used – also that the situation was 'Taken out of my hands'. When asked how they felt about these reactions there was again ambivalence.

> At one level [I was happy with that] because it isn't appropriate for a family who are under strain to have to make additional appointments to see the GP just to keep the GP involved . . . but in another way it feels very odd actually because you are aware that this traumatic event is going on, and months go by . . . I don't want to make more work for anybody really, if the family are happy they are getting what they need elsewhere that's fine. I think the problem is you don't know . . . sometimes afterwards people say I was so alone and nobody asked how it was.

Nine specialists said they were aware that they made the parents 'boycott the GP and local hospitals' and that they should increase contact particularly in preparation for the time when families feel 'suddenly on their own' back in the community after treatment:

> We need to look at putting the trust back into the primary health care team from the parents' point of view.

Only one senior specialist doctor felt that the GP's role did not usefully extend to this period. A consultant offered a more typical view. She was anxious to strengthen links with community care with the initiative coming from the hospital community liaison nurse:

> I think that is how things will develop in the future . . . to provide a link between home and hospital and [the liaison nurse] can help the GP and the health visitor or district nurse, whoever is appropriate, to take over where it is appropriate.

The hospital community liaison service, however, was under tremendous pressure in attempting to meet the families' needs in their homes. There appeared to be little time to spare even to contact the primary health care team except in cases of terminal care. The staff involved in this work did agree, however, about the ideal:

> I think the whole of the community team could be used much more extensively than it is, but it's very time consuming.

Both GPs and specialists appeared to agree that they should work together more closely. Some GPs expressed relief that the emotive and time consuming clinical treatment was taken out of their hands. However, concern was raised about families becoming 'hospital-dependent', believing that 'specialists are the only people who can deal with things'. The majority of health professionals believed that the family doctor had an important contribution to make but were unsure, both about the benefit to their patients and also about how care should be co-ordinated between hospital and community.

THE GP's FUNCTION

The ambivalence on role did not extend to function, for all GPs interviewed felt strongly that they should offer moral support in terms of explanation, interpretation, reassurance, putting things in perspective, listening, understanding, giving the 'space to talk' and express anger and fear within an honest and trusting relationship – in short being 'a professional friend to the family'. The length of time they had known the family and the circumstances of the initial presentation of the disease could influence this relationship for better or worse. Six GPs said that their knowledge of the family put them in an ideal position to deal in particular with 'the family fall-out' – 'to make reasoned judgements for example in the management of collusion'. Four of them had known the family for over ten years seeing them through the birth of the patient and having cared for the parents and grandparents. They felt they were in the best position to have an overall view and review of the families' needs over time.

One GP described her approach highlighting the difference of emphasis necessary in childhood illness in contrast to adult illness; in addition her comments illustrate how a GP's knowledge of the whole family can be of particular benefit in cases of life-threatening illness in children:

> When children are ill the whole family dynamics come into it a lot more than they do in adult illness where by then the family is often down to two people . . . so if a child's illness is causing problems to that child it may reflect itself in other family members, you know somebody else in the family might well come and see me and say, 'You know things are very difficult at home do you think you could have a word with so and so' . . . things like the child might start bed wetting again . . . or other illnesses might be presented as the symptom when in fact the underlying symptom was in fact they had not come to terms with the diagnosis.

Helping families deal with the inevitable fears of uncertainty about whether the cancer would recur, anxieties aroused when similar symptoms to the original illness crop up and the ensuing overprotective behaviour, were aspects which several GPs understood and felt in a position to deal with more immediately than specialists because of their proximity to the family. A GP described a typical situation very vividly:

> It's the availability really you know, that's the only way to help because I think uncertainty leaps up and grabs them from time to time, in an unpredictable manner . . . be prepared to answer questions, to go through it with them whenever they need to.

Whilst GPs felt they could provide a degree of availability, they acknowledged that there was no magic way to resolve the problem of living with uncertainty. They saw their role as 'being there', 'trying to spend that little bit more time' to support, understand and be honest:

If you're going to be truthful about things and say an individual has an 80 per cent chance of being cured ... you naturally leave them in suspense ... that's inevitable.

Another GP said of a mother who frequently brought her child to see him fearing a recurrence of Hodgkin's disease:

As far as we're concerned, if she is very anxious then we're happy to see Amy, that's the first thing. On the other hand we don't like to make a drama of it you know, because we don't want to reinforce anxiety. I want to obviously try and take a little bit of responsibility for accepting that Amy is going to have illnesses just like any other child. So it's a fine line really.

Apart from general support of this kind, GPs said that other practical aspects could be instrumental in helping families cope such as the provision of sick notes for taking time off work, mobilization of extra childcare or social security, treatment of the child's peripheral infections, and dealing with the family's concurrent health care needs which, whilst separate from, should be dealt with within the context of the child's illness.

Whilst specialists generally agreed that GPs should become more involved in the care of these families few were specific about their function at any stage, except for terminal care if the family chose for their child to die at home. One candid reply from a specialist in answer to a question about the possibility of more communication with GPs was:

We send letters ... I don't know how to involve them more ... it's sort of we look after these patients and it's one less for them to worry about.

However another more senior doctor, when asked about a role if the child were in remission, said it was important for the GP to re-establish the relationship, to offer a different perspective from the hospital – 'to take them back into a normal way of life'. GPs themselves placed more emphasis on a **continuing** role through the stages of the child's illness than the specialists. They identified their contribution in three main areas:

- knowledge and awareness of individual family dynamics;
- availability to offer support with living with uncertainty;
- mobilization of local resources to enable easier adjustment to return to 'normal' life within the community.

At whatever stage GPs were involved, however, the predominant view was that their role, though minor during the stages of diagnosis and treatment, was important because 'we have the family for the rest of the time'.

THE RELATIONSHIP OF THE GP TO SPECIALIST CARERS

GPs praised the promptness and quality of information received by letter from the specialist unit particularly at the time of diagnosis. Several emphasized the importance of receiving this information quickly when dealing with the family's questions – 'questions which they may be afraid to ask at hospital, especially initially 'til the relationship with the hospital develops'. They also agreed that the expertise of the consultants and quality of care that families received, particularly the support given in terms of readily available and honest communication of facts regarding diagnosis, prognosis and treatment were of a high standard and surpassed those received by their adult cancer patients:

> Adults with cancer I think the ... information base is much more fragmented, they are referred to different consultants and the counselling they are given is totally inadequate ... if we had a child in a similar situation to that it would be very difficult for us to deal with.

GPs, however, felt excluded once the diagnosis had been made:

> They get to hospital and things get taken out of your hands ... the bandwagon rolls on and together they sort it out, everything becomes hospital focused.

Yet several felt that maintaining contact with the specialists and keeping up to date with the child's progress would help them support the family better and strengthen relationships which could be important for the future. How to effect this, however, appeared difficult. The difficulties divided mainly into two categories – practical and attitudinal.

Practical Factors

The practical factors were mostly associated with pressure on the time available to already hard-pressed health professionals. On the one hand, GPs suggested the specialists should 'steer the family in the direction of the GP more' and, on the other, specialists said the GPs were difficult to contact and the initiative should come from them. The distance involved was another factor raised preventing closer communication. Whilst specialist staff said that GPs were encouraged to come to the regional centre whenever they wished to visit their patients, this was clearly a major problem for those whose patients were up to 80 miles away from their local community. When the child was at home, however, one consultant believed that the role of the primary care team could be greater where a long distance was involved:

> In the active phase of treatment ... we might ask the primary care team to go and sort of assess the situation and clear things up as soon as the child is ill if we're not clear exactly what is going on.

Attitudinal

Practical objections to closer communication can mask difficulties which derive from attitudes about the role and function of professional carers from different disciplines. The respondent quoted above did not see the primary care team as having significant involvement in the care of patients **after** the treatment stage, when they were in remission:

> We have a much higher interest level in our long term survivors ... we want to keep our records up to date, so we tend to see our outpatients six-monthly and so I don't see that as a major role for the primary care team.

The assumption of a 'much higher interest level' appears to undervalue the continuing role and function of the family doctor and lends support to the view of one GP who felt that the attitude of many specialists hindered closer contact between them:

> One difficulty is that hospital doctors think GPs are wallies ... there is this thing that we won't involve the GP because he won't understand. I would like the hospital doctors to sometimes ring us up and help by telling us what is going on, and also to tell the family go to your GP, because some-times hospital doctors deal with the family problems as well, because they feel they are in a better position to do it and actually it detracts from our relationship with the family which may be very important later on.

This respondent was not alone in wanting more **personal** contact with the specialist unit. One GP said 'a voice on the phone would help', another 'outreach into the community, actually coming to see us and talk about it'. It was recognized, however, that the reality of working within a multiprofessional framework is rarely straightforward – the GP, who suggested specialists should take the initiative and 'steer the family in the direction of their GP more', later qualified his comment:

> I have some interest in [paediatric oncology], but I'm sure a lot of GPs would throw up their hands in horror at the thought of dealing with [it] in the community.

But need they be horrified? The families (page 107) said they wanted 'just someone to talk to' about their feelings, about how to get back to normal, how to cope with the uncertainty of whether their child would survive or have a relapse. GPs (page 98) said that they felt their main role was to support the whole family. Given the expressed needs of the family and the willingness of GPs to be involved, it should be possible to promote collaboration between the specialists and the primary health care team. This would require that each accepted the other's complementary role to reduce pressure on available time and resources.

One GP suggested a named keyworker, who could be from the primary health care team or the specialist unit, perhaps chosen by the family:

> ... who routinely informs everybody on progress ... who takes on that sort of sustaining role in an ongoing situation ... so that you know **that** patient's needs are being looked after somewhere at any one time and you are not left wondering.

The respondent claimed this structured approach worked well where they used it with 'long term psychiatric and social cases' and speculated that it could be appropriate for all patients with serious, life-threatening conditions. Additional benefits, she suggested, would be that the family would know who to go to first if they felt desperate and professional carers would be clearer about the allocation of responsibility and time in a situation of competing priorities and possible overlap or duplication of care.

CONCLUSIONS

A diagnosis of childhood cancer hits a family with an explosive force with the ill child at its epicentre, the ripples of distress extending to each member of the family and beyond, to relatives, friends, neighbours and frequently the whole community. The professional carers, both GPs and specialists, found that working in this field was particularly distressing because of the youth of the patient, the sense of helplessness in dealing with parents' anxieties in the face of aggressive treatment with no guarantee of cure, and the severity of impact on the whole family especially if the outcome were terminal. They also stressed the lack of time available to cover all areas of need.

Taking these factors into account it would seem logical to co-ordinate resources to help deal with the multiple effects of childhood cancer. The specialists' role should focus on the disease and the ill child and extend outwards as far as resources allow. The primary health care team can contribute greatly to helping families cope with what are peripheral effects at the time of diagnosis, but their role will become more central as the transition is made from hospital to home and local community. If they have been involved to a degree initially, rather than 'bypassed', they are likely to be more effective at a later stage.

Whilst GPs felt they had an important role to play and specialists were mostly wanting them to have a greater degree of involvement, in practice there was no structure to co-ordinate care. GPs appeared to accept a passive role unless they were called on for terminal care.

A more important dichotomy was found between the perceptions of professional carers and family respondents. Those families who, in the eyes of the health professionals, were 'coping well' were those where the child had responded to treatment. Yet the families revealed that one of the hardest aspects to cope with was living with the uncertainty of their child's survival. Some family members seem to slip between the supporting arms of both specialist and primary health care teams. It is possible that nominating a keyworker from the primary health care team who would liaise closely with the specialist team from the time of diagnosis, and who would co-ordinate (rather than control) care would help give a structure to the care of the whole family. The most appropriate professional, given the individual family history, could then be harnessed so that each member of the family receives appropriate intervention at times of greatest vulnerability and the onus of care is shared.

Without a structure to endorse the principle of multidisciplinary co-operation, deficits in effectiveness and continuity are likely to occur. Further investigation is needed to test a more structured approach to supporting those who live through the experience of childhood cancer and attempt to cope with repercussions which can affect the rest of their lives.

The Way Forward

When a diagnosis of childhood cancer is made there are wide ranging repercussions, not only within the family but also on those who care for them. Although the number of families concerned in this study is small, nevertheless themes have emerged so strongly that it is suggested here that lessons can be learned for the future.

EFFECT ON NORMAL LIFE

The results of this study show that the overall effect on normal life has been seen to be negative for most families, in spite of some secondary gains. This is especially true for mothers who appear to carry a major role in handling the difficult time around diagnosis. Where the extended family is involved, these negative feelings continue, with grandmothers being particularly affected.

These negative effects on normal life could be seen to be a reaction to a difficult diagnosis and yet, in the retrospective group where all patients were in good remission, these negative feelings are considerably stronger than for the prospective group, especially for the patients themselves. The perceived threat, of a return of cancer, clearly leaves feelings of uncertainty which continue to affect normal life.

RELATIONSHIPS

Relationships both within and outside the family are obviously affected when a child has cancer, although for some families the diagnosis brings relationships closer. For some, the worry will be a factor in driving them apart. Children within the family are particularly affected by the nature of the relationships between their parents, patients taking the responsibility for the break up of a marriage, or siblings feeling that somehow they are responsible for what is happening.

What has been shown in relationship terms, however, is the very perceptive nature of children – whether they are the patient trying to protect parents from their worries, or the siblings who often notice much more than their parents in terms of the effect of the illness on the child. This is particularly shown by the sibling in the prospective study who was well aware of how his sister was reacting to a brain tumour and facial paralysis when he said:

She looked pretty sad ... she was thinking ... whether we liked her or not.

This same sibling was also very perceptive about his sister's reaction to her facial paralysis in that he had noted her in the bathroom looking in the mirror and trying to put her face straight on the paralysed side. This happened in a family where the parents felt that the patient had adapted very well to her diagnosis and the resultant disfigurement.

COMING HOME

Although coming home was on the whole a happy occasion for many patients there were again negative elements particularly in terms of individuals, who were well, finding the concept of cancer particularly hard to handle. A major problem here has been seen to be the patient's awareness of the difficulties in that even at 7 years old a child was protecting his parents from the knowledge of his concerns.

The difficulty of a child with cancer coming back into the family is amplified when they return to school and it does seem to be obvious from this study that teachers are not very well prepared to handle a child coming back to school after a diagnosis of cancer. Conversely they are shown to be very thoughtful when a child is first diagnosed, in mounting prayers for the child and family and collecting to send the child presents in hospital, but when the child returns they seem ill equipped to deal with teasing of the patient by other children, or in working out a satisfactory arrangement for the child to catch up with his or her school work.

Another problem in coming home is where there is any change in physical appearance such as hair loss when chemotherapy has been the treatment of choice or disfigurement if caused by the tumour. It is little wonder that children reported feeling that the cancer had made them tougher individuals than they had been before.

REMISSION

Feeling better also brings its own problems. The overall impression has been that the families in the study were all left feeling that the sword of Damocles (Eisenberg, 1981) was hanging over their heads. This was true for the retrospective as well as the prospective study. Being off treatment, having no further blood tests, feeling well, and taking up a normal life, did not appear to take away the fear of recurrence.

The fear of a return of the tumour appeared to be a well kept secret in most families. Each family member would describe his or her own particular fears but would not necessarily have shared those fears with other family members. This was particularly true of the patients in their desire to protect those that they loved from knowing of their own concerns.

These fears of recurrence had an effect on the attitudes towards follow up visits to outpatients for, although many patients found these reassuring and not too worrying if they did not include blood checks, they were however a reminder to others of the fact that cancer had been a part of their life and would always affect the way that they felt overall. A diagnosis of cancer in children as described by family members in this study suggest that even in good remission there are long lasting effects and changes in the lives of both the patients, their immediate family and, if they were very involved, the extended family.

CARERS

It has been shown that childhood cancer affects all family members but in many different ways. It also has been shown to affect those who care for those families, both in hospital and in the community. This extends from the consultant who said that parents did not require a weepy doctor and who then described how if a child relapsed she would cry, to transient staff who found dealing with children who had cancer extraordinarily difficult in emotional terms.

The major problem for the carers however appeared to be in the area of responsibility; when a child has cancer the hospital takes responsibility for that child and family members to the extent that the family can contact the hospital immediately if the child is at home and anything goes wrong. This leaves the GP feeling excluded from the family. Such exclusion is often complete unless the child is dying – when the GP will be brought in, often at the last minute, feeling very vulnerable and ignorant of the pattern of the child's disease.

THE FUTURE

Although many of the negative elements of childhood cancer are inevitable, many of the problems described in this study could be avoided with some thought and care and better use of resources. Most parents, for example, felt that the time of diagnosis was particularly difficult and the 'how' of learning of the seriousness of their child's illness was not always well handled.

Within the family it became obvious that the encouragement of open communication between family members would have decreased feelings of guilt and anger in all members of the family and certainly would have decreased the sense of responsibility and role reversal that was identified in many of the patients.

There also appears to be a role for better education of those involved with children who have cancer, including both family members, teachers, and members of the public.

Finally it could be seen that the role of professional carers had not been clearly defined between care offered by hospital and in the community.

SUPPORT OF FAMILIES

The time at which families are seen to be in most need of support is at diagnosis yet there is little evidence that doctors are taught to give bad news in a sensitive way. (Faulkner *et al.*, 1995) found that, after brief training, doctors who had been very concerned about their inability to break bad news sensitively improved in the way that they gave the bad news message. However, very few in the group had the skills to 'pick up the pieces' after breaking bad news. Most doctors in the study went on to talk to patients and relatives about what they would do about the problem rather than finding out what impact the news had had.

For patients and relatives to be supported at a time of family crisis, medical education must change to include teaching of effective interactive skills, particularly breaking bad news and the identification of immediate and subsequent psychological concerns.

If families are going to adapt to the life crisis of cancer, particularly in a child, they should be offered ongoing support ideally from a member of the health care team. Many parents stressed the need to talk or to be counselled, for example:

The one thing I needed at the time was just having someone to listen to me.

This suggests a clear role within the community in the aftermath of a diagnosis of childhood cancer, and suggests the need for better communication between hospital and community.

A study is currently underway in which practice nurses are taught the skills of working with families so that when a child is diagnosed with a life-threatening illness the practice nurse can work with the family to support them. This would include adequate and relevant information and the identification of psychological concerns. If such a nurse were assigned to a family as a named person at the outset of disease, then the family would know where to turn if things became difficult or if they found that they were not coping. This does not mean taking over the role of other family members in terms of mutual support but does mean working with all family members.

COMMUNICATION

Encouraging open communication

A practice nurse assigned to a family could help to develop open communication within the family and so decrease the risk of collusion. Too often, in an attempt to save a loved one from pain, individuals will keep problems to themselves and minimize any difficulties that they are having. It often takes someone outside the family to help the individual to look at the costs of collusion, and to negotiate the more open approach that will allow individual family members to share their concerns in an open way. Where this did happen as a result of the illness as in the adolescent boy who felt that his sister's illness had brought him much more into his parents' trust, there are obvious benefits both in terms of family members knowing how each other are feeling, but also in terms of siblings feeling valued by their parents in that they are involved in family discussions – perhaps for the first time. What cannot be assumed is that this change will take place without intervention.

Communication between health professionals

If families are to have better support both at the time of diagnosis and during the period of adjustment then there must be better communication between hospital and community. If a practice nurse or another member of the community health care team is assigned to a family, it could be that that individual also had a liaison role with the hospital during the period of the child's illness.

One problem with this proposed solution is the time resource involved. This would have to be negotiated at both community and ward level. However, if this were to take place then the family would feel better supported in that someone would be working with them. This would be instead of putting the onus for getting back to the hospital in times of problems on a family member – usually the mother. There would also be the advantage of the liaison person feeding back to the GP so that there was no longer a feeling of being sidelined when a child was having treatment for a life-threatening disease.

Such liaison between hospital and home will not happen overnight. The hospital staff in the study felt very strongly that, once they take on the care and treatment of a child, that is their responsibility until that child is in remission and beyond. What is required is negotiation between hospital and community personnel to agree the best way forward in the best interests of the child and other family members.

THE TEACHERS

From this study the teacher's role was seen to be very important in easing a child back into normal life. Yet there were problems. Those same teachers who demonstrated the support of the school at the time of diagnosis and first illness, seemed ill equipped to help that child to re-enter school life. This is not surprising given that teachers are not taught in their curricula to handle illness, or a life-threatening diagnosis.

An annual event in Sheffield called 'Gone Forever' is held for teachers to help them to deal with death and dying in the family. This initiative was mounted by Hallam University and Sheffield Area Bereavement Forum. Each year this over-subscribed event highlights the difficulty of the average teacher in handling life-threatening disease and its aftermath.

It is suggested here that part of preparation for teachers should be the handling of illness within a family and the effect it can have on family relationships and a child's ability to handle his or her school work. This should include attention to siblings who may be disorganized by the illness of a brother or sister. Teachers also need to know how to handle teasing when a child suffers a physical change as a result of serious illness.

Attention is required too for planning realistic 'catching up' programmes. One child in the study had a personal tutor during this period which seemed not only to help the child with school work but gave a very necessary boost to confidence.

One way in which the child's re-entry into school could be enhanced would be if children in the school were prepared for any physical disfigurement, such as loss of hair, and helped to understand how **they** would feel if they were coming back to school looking different from when they had last been there. Again teachers would require skills to motivate children in this positive way and it is suggested here that those skills should be part of every teacher's preparation to teach.

THE PUBLIC

For most people cancer remains a fear provoking word that equates with death. In this situation most people simply do not know what to say (Buckman, 1988), and so they avoid the person and their family. Children in such circumstances may revert to teasing and making unpleasant jokes. The media tends to reinforce the negative message about cancer, and patients and their families identify with this message and often do not understand that the negative behaviour they see from those around them is born of ignorance and embarrassment rather than of anything else.

There is a positive side to the cancer scene. Fewer people die of cancer than of heart disease, and childhood cancer has very good recovery rates overall. In spite of this, in the study described here, even the retrospective group in good remission continued to fear the return of their cancer.

If children with cancer are to be reinstated in the community after their treatment is over and when they are feeling better, then the public must be educated in terms of what to expect from the child, and how to help that child fit in with society.

When a child has cancer, this may bring problems for the whole family. All family members may require support from those around them including the health professionals who care for the family and friends and teachers at school. This support is only possible with improved education of health professionals, teachers, and the public, so that the needs of any individual within the family are accurately identified and sensitively met from the period of diagnosis through to recovery or death.

REFERENCES

Buckman, R. (1988) *I Don't Know What to Say*. Macmillan Press, Basingstoke.

Eisenberg, L. (1981) The Foreword. In *The Damocles Syndrome*, (eds G.P. Koocher and J.E. Malley) McGraw-Hill, New York, pp. xi–xv.

Faulkner, A., O'Keeffe, C., Argent, J. and Jones, A. (1995) *Improving the skills of doctors in breaking bad news* (in press).

Useful addresses

ACT (Care of families where a child has a life-threatening illness)
The Institute of Child Health, 65 St Michael's Hill, Bristol BS2 8BJ.
Tel. 01272 221556.

BACUP (Cancer support and information)
121/123 Charterhouse Street, London EC1M 6AA.
Tel. 0171 608 1661.

CALL (Childhood cancer and leukaemia link)
20 Haywood, Bracknell, Berks RG12 4WG.
Tel. 01344 423635.

Cancerlink (Emotional support and information)
17 Britannia Street, London WC1X 9JN.
Tel. 0171 833 2451.

Children's Cancer Fund (Children's cancer care)
262 The Broadway, Wimbledon, London SW19 1SB.
Tel. 0181 543 5979.

Childhood Cancer Research Group (Research)
University of Oxford, 57 Woodstock Road, Oxford OX2 6HJ.
Tel. 01865 310030.

Christian Lewis Trust (Support for families where a child has cancer)
PO Box 2, Swansea SA1 1PP.
Tel. 01792 363888.

CLIC UK (Cancer and leukaemia in childhood trust)
4 Wimpole Street, London W1.
Tel. 0171 637 4005

Malcolm Sargent Cancer Fund for Children (Welfare)
14 Abingdon Road, London W8 6AF.
Tel. 0171 937 4548.

Rainbow Centre for Children with Cancer and Life-Threatening Illness (Therapeutic support and complementary therapies)
PO Box 604, Bristol BS99 1SW.
Tel. 01272 736228.

Index